LIGHT SWORD
MOVEMENT THERAPY

LIGHT SWORD MOVEMENT THERAPY

Igniting Your Inner Warrior Through Light Sword Mixed Martial Arts

SIFU EDWARD ARMSTRONG

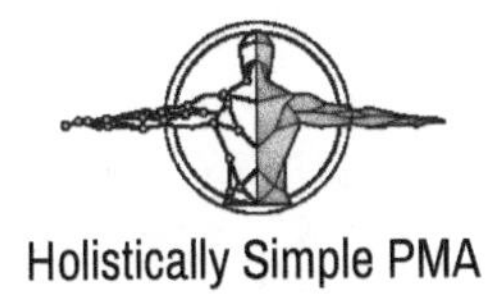

Holistically Simple PMA

CONTENTS

Introduction vii

1 CHAPTER ONE 1

2 CHAPTER TWO 15

3 CHAPTER THREE 37

4 CHAPTER FOUR 72

5 CHAPTER FIVE 105

6 CHAPTER SIX 126

7 CHAPTER SEVEN 154

8 CHAPTER EIGHT 185

9 CHAPTER NINE 210

Acknowledgments 227
About The Author 229

INTRODUCTION

The Unexplored Crisis in Modern Martial Arts

Recognizing the Stagnation in Traditional Practices
- Defining the crisis: Lack of innovation in martial arts
- Stories of practitioners feeling uninspired
- Costs: Declining interest and loss of potential benefits
- Actions: Embrace a new perspective on martial arts

Welcome to a journey of transformation, a journey that begins with recognizing a crisis in the world of martial arts. You're about to embark on an exploration that challenges the status quo, breaks down barriers, and unveils a path to rejuvenation and passion in martial arts. This journey is not just about learning a new discipline; it's about rekindling the fire within, about igniting a spark in a field that has long been stagnating in traditional practices.

As we stand today, martial arts face an unspoken crisis – a crisis of innovation, or rather, the lack thereof. Traditional martial arts, with their rich heritage and time-tested techniques, have been cornerstones of discipline, self-defense, and physical fitness. But let's face it, the world is evolving, and so are our needs, our interests, and our ways of engaging with physical disciplines.

I've encountered countless martial arts practitioners, each with their unique story, but a common thread emerges – a sense of being uninspired, of yearning for something more, something that resonates with the pulse of today's fast-paced, ever-changing world. These stories are not just anecdotes; they are a reflection of a widespread sentiment. Think about it – when was the last time you felt truly exhilarated in your martial arts practice? When did you last feel that your training was not just a routine but a thrilling, fulfilling adventure?

This stagnation comes at a cost. We are witnessing a declining interest in traditional martial arts, especially among the younger generation. They seek excitement, relevance, and engagement – elements that current traditional practices may not fully provide. This decline is not just a loss of numbers; it's a loss of potential – potential for physical betterment, mental discipline, and the growth of a vibrant, diverse martial arts community.

But what if I told you there's a way to turn this around? What if there's a perspective that breathes new life into martial arts, making it relevant, exciting, and deeply engaging once again? This is where we introduce the concept of innovation in martial arts, a concept that's at the heart of this book.

Imagine integrating the time-honored techniques of traditional martial arts with the dynamic, visually stunning world of lightsaber combat. Picture a discipline that combines physical rigor with mental agility, and strategic thinking with creative expression. This is not just about wielding a lightsaber; it's about embracing a new perspective on martial arts, one that revitalizes its essence and makes it resonate with our modern lifestyle.

As we step into this new era, it's crucial to understand that embracing change in martial arts isn't just about adding a new layer to your physical routine but redefining what it means to you. It's about seeing martial arts not just as a set of movements and techniques but as a living, breathing entity that grows, evolves, and resonates with the spirit of its time.

Think about the young person who walks into a dojo, eyes full of curiosity, seeking skills and an experience that resonates with their understanding of the world. Or consider the long-time practitioner, skilled in traditional forms, yet searching for something to rekindle their passion, to connect their practice with the vibrant energy of the modern world. These are not isolated cases; they are signs of a widespread craving for innovation, for a martial arts practice that's as dynamic and multifaceted as the world we live in.

The cost of ignoring this craving for innovation is not just a decline in interest. It's a missed opportunity for martial arts to evolve, to contribute meaningfully to our physical and mental well-being in a world where these aspects are increasingly vital. We are at a crossroads where the choice to innovate can lead us to a future where martial arts continue to inspire, challenge, and captivate.

How, then, do we embrace this new perspective? The answer lies in openness – openness to new ideas, new techniques, and new forms of expression within martial arts. It lies in acknowledging that the essence of martial arts – discipline, strength, strategy, and self-improvement – can be preserved and even enhanced through innovative practices.

Lightsaber MMA stands at the forefront of this innovative wave. It's a discipline that challenges the norms, pushes boundaries, and opens up a world of possibilities. It combines the grace and discipline of traditional martial arts with the energy and excitement of wielding a lightsaber, creating an experience that is both deeply rooted and exhilaratingly fresh.

Imagine the exhilaration of mastering a lightsaber, of engaging in combat that's not just physically demanding but also mentally stimulating. Picture yourself being part of a community that's diverse, vibrant, and supportive, where each member is on a journey of personal growth and discovery. This is not a distant dream; it's a tangible reality that lightsaber MMA offers.

In this book, we'll navigate this exciting landscape together. We'll explore how lightsaber MMA can transform your practice, enhance your physical and mental capabilities, and connect you with a community of like-minded individuals. We'll dive into stories of transformation and growth, showcasing the profound impact of this innovative discipline. And most importantly, we'll outline actionable steps that you can take to start your journey in lightsaber MMA, to be part of this exciting new chapter in martial arts.

In the pages that follow, we will delve into this new world. We'll explore how innovation can bridge the gap between traditional martial arts and the needs of today's practitioners. We'll hear stories of transformation, of individuals who found new passion and purpose in their practice. And most importantly, we'll discover actions you can take to be part of this exciting new chapter in the world of martial arts.

So, are you ready to embark on this journey? Are you ready to embrace a new perspective and rediscover your passion for martial arts? Let's dive in!

CHAPTER ONE

Igniting the Spark:
The Need for Innovation in Martial Arts

Identifying the Gap in Martial Arts Training
*   - Defining the gap: Traditional vs. modern needs*
*   - Examples of outdated methods*
*   - Benefits of adopting innovative approaches*
*   - Actions: Steps to integrate new practices*

Subsection: Identifying the Gap in Martial Arts Training

1. Defining the Gap: Traditional vs. Modern Needs

In our quest to understand the evolving landscape of martial arts, it's essential to confront a critical reality – the growing gap between traditional practices and modern needs. This gap is more than just a difference in techniques or teaching methods; it represents a divergence in expectations, aspirations, and relevance in today's world.

Traditional martial arts, with their deep roots in ancient cultures and philosophies, have provided a foundation of discipline, respect, and physical prowess for centuries. These arts have taught us the value of patience, the importance of ritual, and the power of mastery through repetition. But let's ask ourselves: Are these time-honored practices in sync with the pace, challenges, and mindset of our modern world? The world today moves at a breakneck speed, fueled by rapid technological advancements and a constant influx of information. People seek activities that not only provide physical benefits but also offer mental stimulation, emotional engagement, and a sense of immediate accomplishment.

The traditional dojo, with its focus on repetitive drills and adherence to long-established forms, might not fully cater to these contemporary desires. The younger generation, especially, raised in a digital age, often looks for practices that are more dynamic, more immediately gratifying, and more in tune with their everyday experiences. They yearn for a martial arts experience that is not just about learning movements and techniques, but about experiencing a journey that is mentally stimulating, emotionally rewarding, and closely aligned with their lifestyle.

Moreover, the traditional one-size-fits-all approach to training often overlooks the diversity of learning styles and physical capabilities. In contrast, modern martial arts enthusiasts seek personalized training experiences that recognize and adapt to individual differences. They value environments where they can express themselves freely, where innovation and creativity are not just allowed but encouraged.

Let's consider the physical aspects as well. Traditional martial arts, while effective in developing certain skills, may not always provide a comprehensive workout that meets today's fitness standards. People now look for training that challenges them in a variety of ways — cardiovascular endurance, strength, flexibility, and agility — all in one session. The modern martial artist seeks a practice that is as diverse and multifaceted as their lives.

So, what does bridging this gap look like? It involves integrating the discipline and depth of traditional martial arts with the energy and innovation of modern practices. It's about creating a fusion that respects and preserves the essence of traditional martial arts while infusing it with new life and relevance. This fusion leads to a form of martial arts that is not only physically comprehensive but also mentally and emotionally stimulating.

In our exploration, we'll see how practices like lightsaber MMA embody this fusion. They offer a holistic approach that aligns with the fast-paced, diverse, and technology-driven world we live in. By embracing this new perspective, we can make martial arts more accessible, more engaging, and more relevant to people from all walks of life.

This understanding of the gap between traditional and modern needs is not just an observation; it's a call to action. It's an invitation to evolve, to innovate, and to reimagine what martial arts can be. It's about taking the timeless values of traditional martial arts and translating them into a language that resonates with the modern practitioner.

As we delve deeper into this journey, keep an open mind. Consider how the principles and practices of traditional martial arts can be adapted to meet the needs of today's world. Think about how you, as a practitioner, can contribute to this evolution. The future of martial arts is not set in stone; it's a path waiting to be forged, a narrative waiting to be written. Let's embark on this journey together, with the spirit of innovation guiding our way.

2. Examples of Outdated Methods

In our exploration of martial arts and its evolution, it's crucial to understand specific examples of outdated methods in traditional practices. These methods, while once groundbreaking, may no longer fully serve the needs of contemporary practitioners. It's not about dismissing these methods; rather, it's about recognizing where and how we can infuse new life into them.

- Rigid Training Routines

  Traditional martial arts often emphasize rigid, unvarying training routines. These routines, which include repetitive drills and set forms (katas or poomsae), are designed to instill discipline and precision. However, in today's dynamic world, such rigidity can be limiting. It doesn't always allow for the creativity and adaptability that modern life demands. The younger generation, accustomed to a more flexible and interactive learning environment, may find these rigid routines monotonous and disengaging.

- One-Size-Fits-All Approach

  The traditional martial arts teaching methodology often follows a one-size-fits-all approach. This method doesn't account for the diverse learning styles, physical abilities, and personal goals of students. In contrast, modern learners seek a more personalized experience that acknowledges their unique strengths and challenges. They thrive in environments where training is tailored to their individual needs, allowing for a more inclusive and effective learning experience.

- Limited Focus on Holistic Fitness

   While traditional martial arts excel in developing specific skills like balance and coordination, they sometimes lack a comprehensive approach to physical fitness. Modern fitness standards emphasize a combination of strength training, cardiovascular endurance, flexibility, and agility. Traditional methods, focusing primarily on technique and form, may not provide the holistic physical conditioning that is increasingly sought after in today's health-conscious society.

- Overemphasis on Tradition and Ceremony

   Tradition and ceremony are integral to traditional martial arts, imbuing the practice with a sense of history and reverence. However, an overemphasis on these aspects can sometimes overshadow practical training and application. Especially in self-defense training, there's a need for more pragmatic, real-world scenarios that prepare students for unpredictable situations they might encounter outside the dojo.

- Insufficient Engagement with Modern Technology

   In an age where technology plays a central role in our lives, traditional martial arts often lag in integrating modern technological tools. This gap is evident in training methods, communication, and engagement strategies. Today's practitioners, especially the younger generation, are accustomed to and expect a certain level of technological engagement, whether it's through online training modules, virtual reality simulations, or interactive learning apps.

- Lack of Cross-Disciplinary Training

  Traditional martial arts disciplines tend to focus intensely on their specific style, often at the expense of cross-disciplinary training. However, the modern martial artist values a more versatile skill set. They recognize the benefits of integrating techniques and principles from various martial arts forms, understanding that such cross-disciplinary training leads to a better-rounded and adaptable combat skill set.

It's about evolving the practice to make it more relevant, engaging, and effective for today's practitioners. This evolution isn't about discarding the old; it's about enriching it with new insights and approaches. As we continue through this book, remember that every step towards innovation in martial arts is a step towards keeping this ancient art form alive and thriving in our modern world.

Let me share with you the story of Alex, a close friend and martial arts enthusiast, whose journey vividly illustrates the transformative power of embracing innovation in martial arts. Alex's story is not just about a shift in training style; it's a tale of rediscovery, passion, and the rekindling of a lost spark.

Alex had been practicing traditional martial arts since childhood. He was dedicated, disciplined, and deeply respectful of the art. Over the years, he achieved considerable proficiency, and his life seemed inextricably linked to the dojo's rhythmic routines. Yet, as time passed, Alex began to feel a sense of disconnection. The once exhilarating practice had become a mere routine. The katas and drills, once challenging, now felt overly familiar, almost mechanical. He found himself going through the motions, with the passion that once fueled his practice reduced to a flickering flame.

This sense of disconnection troubled Alex deeply. Martial arts were a part of his identity, but the joy and excitement that once drove him were waning. It was during this period of introspection that Alex stumbled upon a demonstration of lightsaber MMA at a local fitness expo. Initially skeptical, he watched, intrigued by the fluidity, the dynamism, and the unmistakable energy of the practitioners. It was unlike anything he had seen in traditional dojos – it was traditional martial arts but with an electrifying twist.

Driven by curiosity, Alex decided to attend a lightsaber MMA workshop. From the moment he held the lightsaber, something shifted within him. The familiar principles of balance, coordination, and discipline were all there, but there was something new – an element of creativity, of expressiveness that traditional martial arts had not offered him. The lightsaber felt like an extension of himself, yet it challenged him in ways he had not anticipated. Each movement, each combat scenario, required not just physical skill but strategic thinking and adaptability.

As Alex delved deeper into lightsaber MMA, the lost spark of passion was rekindled. He found himself eagerly awaiting each training session, experimenting with movements, and engaging with the vibrant community of practitioners. The blend of tradition and innovation in lightsaber MMA resonated with him, bridging the gap between the martial arts discipline he respected and the modern, dynamic approach he craved.

Alex's journey with lightsaber MMA became a journey of self-discovery. He rediscovered his passion for martial arts, but more importantly, he discovered new dimensions of himself – his creativity, his adaptability, and his capacity for joy in practice. He often shares that lightsaber MMA didn't just change his training; it transformed his perspective on martial arts and life.

Alex's story is a testament to the power of embracing innovation in martial arts. It reminds us that sometimes, to rekindle our passion, we need to step out of our comfort zones and explore new horizons. His journey from disconnection to rediscovery is an inspiration, illustrating that the heart of martial arts lies not in rigid adherence to tradition but in the spirit of continuous learning and evolution.

3. Benefits of Adopting Innovative Approaches

In our transformative journey through the world of martial arts, embracing innovation isn't just a choice; it's a necessity to stay relevant and effective. When we adopt innovative approaches in martial arts, like integrating lightsaber MMA, we're not just tweaking a training routine – we're opening doors to a multitude of benefits that resonate with our modern lifestyle and aspirations. Let's delve deeper into these benefits:

- Enhanced Physical Fitness and Versatility
  One of the most significant benefits of adopting innovative approaches in martial arts is the enhanced physical fitness and versatility it offers. Lightsaber MMA, for instance, isn't just about learning to handle a lightsaber; it's a complete workout regime. It amalgamates the discipline of traditional martial arts with the agility and cardiovascular intensity required in lightsaber combat. This combination ensures that practitioners get a more diverse and comprehensive physical workout than what traditional forms may offer. It's about engaging different muscle groups, improving cardiovascular health, and enhancing overall physical agility and strength.

- Mental and Cognitive Benefits
  In today's fast-paced world, mental agility and cognitive

flexibility are as important as physical strength. Innovative martial arts practices like lightsaber MMA challenge not just the body but also the mind. They require strategic thinking, quick decision-making, and mental adaptability, much like a game of physical chess. This mental engagement helps sharpen cognitive abilities, enhances problem-solving skills, and improves concentration. These are skills that extend far beyond the dojo – they are essential in every aspect of our daily lives.

- Emotional Growth and Resilience

   Martial arts have always been a pathway to emotional growth and resilience, but innovative approaches take this one step further. Practices like lightsaber MMA offer an expressive outlet that combines physical exertion with emotional expression. The thrill and excitement that come with learning something new and dynamic like lightsaber combat can be immensely satisfying and empowering. This emotional engagement helps build confidence, reduce stress, and promote a sense of well-being. It's about channeling energy positively, managing emotions effectively, and developing a resilient mindset.

- Fostering Creativity and Innovation

   By stepping into innovative practices, we're also fostering a spirit of creativity and innovation in martial arts. Lightsaber MMA, with its blend of traditional and modern elements, encourages practitioners to think outside the box, to be creative in their techniques and strategies. This openness to creativity not only makes training more enjoyable but also inspires continuous improvement and evolution in martial arts techniques and teaching methods.

• Building a Diverse and Inclusive Community

Adopting innovative martial arts practices often leads to the creation of a more diverse and inclusive community. These modern forms of martial arts, with their universal appeal and adaptable nature, attract a wide range of individuals, regardless of age, background, or skill level. This diversity enriches the training experience, as practitioners learn from each other's unique perspectives and experiences. It fosters a sense of community that is supportive, vibrant, and united by a shared passion for martial arts.

• Enhancing Real-World Applicability

In today's world, the applicability of martial arts in real-life scenarios is more crucial than ever. Innovative martial arts practices are often designed with a focus on practicality and real-world relevance. They combine traditional defense techniques with scenarios that mimic real-life confrontations, providing practitioners with skills that are not just theoretically sound but also practically effective.

We are not just learning a new form of martial arts; we are equipping ourselves with skills that are essential for our physical, mental, and emotional well-being in the modern world. We are participating in the evolution of an ancient practice, ensuring that it continues to be relevant, effective, and enriching for generations to come.

4. Actions: Steps to Integrate New Practices

As we embrace the call to innovate in martial arts, the question arises: How do we effectively integrate these new practices into our routine? Transformation requires action, and in this case, it involves a series of strategic steps that can usher in a new era in your martial arts journey. Let's dive into these steps, each designed to guide you toward successfully integrating innovative practices like lightsaber MMA into your martial arts repertoire.

- Cultivate an Open Mindset

  The first step in integrating new practices is to cultivate an open, growth-oriented mindset. Embrace the idea that martial arts are a living, evolving discipline that can benefit from new perspectives. Let go of any preconceived notions that may limit your openness to innovation. Remember, every great martial artist started as a student who was open to learning.

- Research and Explore

  Begin by immersing yourself in the world of innovative martial arts. Research what's out there – read articles, watch videos, and follow experts in the field of lightsaber MMA and other modern martial arts practices. This exploration will not only broaden your understanding but also ignite your curiosity and excitement about the possibilities these new practices offer.

- Connect with Innovators and Practitioners

  Seek out and connect with innovators and practitioners of modern martial arts. Attend workshops, seminars, or classes where these new practices are taught. Engaging with those who are at the forefront of martial arts innovation provides invaluable insights and first-hand experience. It also helps you build a network of like-minded individuals who share your passion for martial arts evolution.

- Start Small and Experiment

   Integration doesn't have to be an all-or-nothing approach. Start small by incorporating elements of innovative practices into your existing routine. It could be as simple as adding a lightsaber MMA drill to your workout or practicing a new technique you learned from a workshop. Experiment with different aspects and observe how they enhance your practice. This gradual approach allows you to adjust and adapt comfortably.

- Reflect and Adapt

   As you experiment with new practices, take time to reflect on your experience. What's working? What's not? How do these new methods enhance your martial arts journey? Use these reflections to adapt your approach. Remember, the goal is to enhance your martial arts practice, making it more engaging, effective, and enjoyable.

- Share and Inspire Others

   Sharing your journey with others can be incredibly rewarding. It not only reinforces your learning but also inspires others to explore new practices. Share your experiences in your dojo, online forums, or social media. Your journey could be the spark that ignites a passion for innovation in someone else.

- Commit to Continuous Learning

    Finally, commit to being a lifelong learner. The world of martial arts is vast and ever-evolving. By staying committed to learning and evolving, you ensure that your practice remains dynamic and fulfilling. Attend regular training sessions, workshops, and seminars. Stay updated on the latest trends and techniques. This commitment to continuous learning is what will keep your martial arts practice vibrant and relevant.

Remember, integrating new practices into your martial arts training is a journey, not a destination. It's about exploring, experimenting, and evolving. It's about taking the best of what the traditional has to offer and enhancing it with the innovation of the modern. This journey is yours to take, and every step you take towards innovation is a step towards a more fulfilling and dynamic martial arts experience.

* * *

Footnotes

Based on the research and expert opinions from Aikido Journal, the following references provide insights into the evolution of martial arts practices from traditional methods to innovative approaches:

1. **The Necessity of Innovation in Classical Martial Arts**: Charles Humphrey, in his article, highlights the lack of innovation and logical progression in classical martial arts training methodologies.

He emphasizes the need for a new perspective that integrates personal research into neuroscience, exercise, and sports science to enhance martial arts training, citing Systema School as an example of effective innovation due to its unique approach1.

2. **Balancing Tradition and Innovation**: Humphrey advises against extreme adherence to traditionalism, noting the importance of understanding the limitations of classical methods and the need for innovation. He cites Bruce Lee as an example of a martial artist who practiced traditional methods before innovating, underscoring that neither extreme traditionalism nor complete rejection of tradition is beneficial1.

3. **Effective Use of Traditional Curriculum**: The traditional curriculum in martial arts, such as the Daito-Ryu system or Aikido schools, is viewed as a tool that can be adapted and used in various ways. Humphrey suggests that traditional kata-based training, with its attention to detail, can be integrated into a broader training approach that includes general physical preparation GPP◇188†source◇.

4. **Cycling Training Modules**: The concept of cycling training modules is proposed as an effective way to program movements into the body, considering the understanding of the nervous system, brain, muscles, and skeleton. This approach is contrasted with the typical methodology in many martial arts schools, where a wide range of techniques is covered without a focused and repetitive approach to reach proficiency1.

5. **Encouragement for Experimentation and Innovation**: Martial arts practitioners are encouraged to explore and innovate beyond the teachings of their old instructors, emphasizing the importance of not being confined to past methods. This mindset fosters a more dynamic and adaptable approach to martial arts training, which is more aligned with contemporary needs and understanding1.

These references underscore the importance of evolving martial arts practices by integrating traditional foundations with innovative approaches. They highlight the necessity of this evolution in the context of modern martial arts training, emphasizing adaptability, continuous learning, and the integration of contemporary scientific understanding into martial arts methodologies.

CHAPTER TWO

The Promise of Lightsaber MMA

Visualizing a New Era of Martial Arts
- Defining the unique blend of lightsaber MMA
- Success stories of transformation
- Benefits: Physical, mental, & community enhancement
- Actions: How to begin your journey in lightsaber MMA

Subsection: Visualizing a New Era of Martial Arts

1. *Defining the Unique Blend of Lightsaber MMA*

Lightsaber Mixed Martial Arts (MMA) represents a groundbreaking fusion in the world of martial arts, seamlessly blending the time-honored traditions of classical combat forms with the futuristic allure and dynamism of lightsaber combat. This unique blend transcends the boundaries of traditional martial arts, offering a new and exhilarating approach to physical fitness, mental agility, and personal expression.

• Integration of Traditional Martial Arts Principles

At its core, lightsaber MMA retains the fundamental principles that have been the cornerstone of traditional martial arts for centuries. These include discipline, respect, precision, and mindfulness. Practitioners of lightsaber MMA engage in routines and exercises that emphasize these values, ensuring that the essence of martial arts is preserved and honored.

• Incorporation of Lightsaber Combat Techniques

What sets lightsaber MMA apart is the incorporation of lightsaber combat techniques. This aspect introduces an element of novelty and excitement, attracting practitioners with its unique blend of choreography and combat strategy. The lightsaber, as a combat tool, requires agility, coordination, and a deep understanding of spatial awareness, adding a new dimension to the martial arts experience.

• Focus on Creativity and Personal Expression

Lightsaber MMA encourages creativity and personal expression. Unlike traditional martial arts, where routines and forms are often rigid and predefined, lightsaber MMA allows practitioners to infuse their personality into their combat style. This freedom of expression makes each practitioner's journey with lightsaber MMA unique and deeply personal.

- Enhanced Physical and Cognitive Engagement

The practice of lightsaber MMA is physically demanding, combining the cardiovascular intensity of high-impact martial arts with the precision and control of traditional forms. Additionally, it engages cognitive functions, requiring practitioners to make quick decisions and strategize in real time during combat simulations and sparring sessions.

- Adaptability and Modern Relevance

Lightsaber MMA stands out for its adaptability and relevance in today's world. It appeals to a wide audience, from avid martial arts enthusiasts to fans of science fiction and fantasy, making it a diverse and inclusive practice. Its modern twist on traditional martial arts makes it particularly appealing to the younger generation, who find in it a connection to contemporary culture and interests.

- Community and Cultural Impact

The practice of lightsaber MMA has given rise to a new community of martial artists. This community is characterized by its inclusivity, shared passion, and mutual respect. The cultural impact of lightsaber MMA extends beyond the dojo, influencing popular media and bringing a fresh perspective to the portrayal of martial arts in contemporary culture.

Lightsaber MMA represents a harmonious blend of tradition and innovation, discipline and creativity, physical prowess and mental agility. It's a discipline that not only offers a comprehensive martial arts experience but also resonates with the aspirations and sensibilities of modern practitioners, making it a vibrant and evolving form of martial arts in the 21st century.

A Profound Moment of Appreciation in Teaching Lightsaber MMA:

There's a moment in teaching that every instructor cherishes – a moment of clarity, a profound realization of the impact their teaching has on others. I experienced one such moment while teaching a lightsaber MMA class, a moment that not only deepened my appreciation for this unique martial art but also reinforced my belief in the power of innovation and adaptation in personal growth and development.

I was leading a diverse group of students through a lightsaber MMA session. The group was varied – some were seasoned martial artists looking to explore something new, while others were complete novices, drawn by the allure of the lightsaber. As the class progressed, I noticed how each student, regardless of their background, was deeply engaged. The energy in the room was electric, a blend of focus, excitement, and a shared sense of adventure.

It was during a sparring session that my moment of profound appreciation came. Two students were engaged in a lightsaber duel – a dance of lights if you will. One was a young woman, hardly in her twenties, a beginner in martial arts but with a natural grace and agility. Her opponent was a middle-aged man, experienced in traditional martial arts but new to the world of lightsaber MMA. The duel was a captivating display of strategy, agility, and respect. Each strike, each parry, was executed with precision and mindfulness.

As I watched them, it struck me – lightsaber MMA was more than just a physical discipline. It was a medium that brought together people from all walks of life, each with their own stories, their battles, and their aspirations. Here, in this dance of lightsabers, age, background, experience – none of it mattered. What mattered was the shared experience, the mutual respect, and the collective pursuit of mastery and self-improvement.

I realized then that what I was teaching was not just a set of techniques or combat strategies. I was facilitating a journey of discovery and growth. Lightsaber MMA, with its unique blend of traditional martial arts principles and the dynamic, creative aspects of lightsaber combat, was helping these students not only improve their physical skills but also develop mentally and emotionally. It was teaching them about adaptability, the importance of mental agility, and the joy of stepping out of their comfort zones.

This moment was a powerful reminder of the unique potential of lightsaber MMA. It underscored the importance of innovation in martial arts – not just for the sake of novelty, but for the profound impact it can have on practitioners. It was a testament to the fact that when we blend the wisdom of the old with the vibrancy of the new, we create something truly extraordinary.

As the class ended and the students left, each carrying their piece of this experience, I stood there, filled with a deep sense of gratitude and purpose. Teaching lightsaber MMA was not just a profession; it was a privilege, an opportunity to impact lives, inspire growth, and be part of a journey that went far beyond the physical dimensions of martial arts.

2. Success Stories of Transformation

The transformative journey of lightsaber MMA practitioners is nothing short of inspiring. These stories are not just about mastering a new form of martial arts; they are about personal growth, confidence-building, and community.

Diverse Stories of Transformation through Lightsaber MMA

1. Sarah's Journey to Empowerment

Sarah was a young professional who struggled with self-confidence and staying fit. She stumbled upon a lightsaber MMA class almost by accident. Initially skeptical, she was quickly captivated by the energy and community spirit. Within months of training, Sarah experienced a remarkable transformation. Her fitness levels soared – she was stronger and more agile, and her endurance had improved significantly. More importantly, wielding the lightsaber made her feel empowered and confident. She described the experience as "liberating." Lightsaber MMA became her avenue for self-expression and empowerment, drastically improving her self-esteem and overall well-being. Sarah's story is a testament to how integrating fun and innovation in exercise can lead to profound personal growth.

1. Mark's Recovery and Renewal

Mark, a former athlete, had fallen out of shape due to a severe injury that shook his confidence and left him disconnected from physical activities. Discovering lightsaber MMA was a turning point in his life. The adaptability of the training allowed him to participate without aggravating his injury. Slowly, he regained his physical strength and confidence.

The strategic and mental aspects of lightsaber combat provided him with a new challenge that rekindled his competitive spirit. Mark shared, "Lightsaber MMA didn't just help me recover physically; it helped me find a part of myself I thought I had lost after the injury." His journey highlights the role of innovative fitness approaches in rehabilitation and mental resilience.

1. Emily's Escape from Monotony

Emily, a middle-aged mother of two, joined a lightsaber MMA class seeking a break from her routine life. She found much more than she bargained for. The classes provided her with an exhilarating escape, offering both physical and mental stimulation. Emily noticed significant improvements in her flexibility and overall fitness. More importantly, lightsaber MMA became her sanctuary – a place where she could release stress and reconnect with herself. "It's my time to just be me, not a mom, not a wife, just me," Emily reflected. Her story is a powerful example of how adopting new, engaging forms of exercise can bring joy and balance to our lives.

1. Liam's Conquest of Anxiety

Liam, a college student, struggled with social anxiety and found it hard to connect with others or participate in group activities. He was drawn to a lightsaber MMA club on campus, intrigued by its inclusive and welcoming environment. Training in lightsaber MMA became a journey of self-discovery for Liam. He not only saw improvements in his physical health but also in his ability to interact and bond with others. The practice sessions became a safe space for him to open up, build confidence, and overcome his anxiety. "Lightsaber MMA gave me a community where I felt accepted and confident enough to be my-self," Liam shared. His experience underscores how innovative activities like lightsaber MMA can foster social connections and improve mental health.

Overcoming Challenges Through Lightsaber Mixed Martial Arts: Inspirational Practitioners' Stories

1. Jake's Triumph over Physical Adversity

Jake's story is one of remarkable resilience and strength. A former marathon runner, he faced a devastating setback after a severe leg injury. The physical limitations imposed by his injury were not just a hindrance to his athletic pursuits; they severely impacted his mental health. When Jake discovered lightsaber MMA, it initially seemed like an unattainable dream. However, the adaptable nature of the practice allowed him to participate at his own pace. Gradually, he regained strength and mobility in his leg. More importantly, lightsaber MMA restored his confidence and gave him a renewed sense of purpose. Jake's journey is a powerful illustration of how innovative practices can aid physical rehabilitation and boost mental resilience.

2. Maria's Battle with Depression

Maria's encounter with lightsaber MMA came at a time when she was battling severe depression. Feeling disconnected and unmotivated, she struggled to find joy in her daily life. Lightsaber MMA, with its unique combination of physical activity and community support, became a lifeline for her. The physical exertion helped in alleviating some of her depressive symptoms, while the sense of accomplishment and belonging she found within the lightsaber MMA community played a crucial role in her mental health recovery. Maria credits lightsaber MMA for helping her regain control of her life, stating, "It's more than a sport; it's a journey to self-recovery."

3. Tom's Conquest of Social Anxiety

Social anxiety had always been a barrier for Tom, preventing him from fully engaging in group activities or forming new relationships. His introduction to lightsaber MMA was a chance encounter – a friend invited him to a class. The inclusive and supportive environment of the lightsaber MMA community was a game-changer for Tom. It provided him with a safe space to interact and connect with others, gradually overcoming his social anxiety. The discipline required in the training also instilled in him a sense of self-confidence that transcended the dojo. Tom's story is a testament to the power of community and the role of martial arts in overcoming mental health challenges.

4. Angela's Journey of Self-Discovery

Angela turned to lightsaber MMA during a period of self-doubt and identity crisis. As a single mother and a career professional, she often felt overwhelmed by the pressures of her responsibilities. Lightsaber MMA offered her an outlet for stress and a platform for personal growth. The training not only helped her stay physically fit but also provided mental clarity. Through mastering the techniques and engaging with the community, Angela discovered inner strength and confidence she never knew she had. She describes lightsaber MMA as "a transformative experience that reshaped my self-perception and taught me the true meaning of empowerment."

Chris's Journey: Finding Solace in Lightsaber MMA

In the realm of transformation and personal growth, Chris's story stands out as a profound testament to the healing power of engaging in innovative practices like lightsaber MMA. Chris, an Army veteran, carried the weight of his experiences from his time in service, battling PTSD which cast a shadow over his everyday life. His journey with lightsaber MMA, however, opened a new chapter of healing and self-discovery, showcasing the incredible resilience of the human spirit.

Chris first encountered lightsaber MMA at a local community center. Initially skeptical, he was drawn to the unique blend of discipline and creativity it offered. The physical aspects of lightsaber MMA were familiar territory – the discipline, the structure, and the focus on physical fitness. But it was the artistry, the fluidity, and the community spirit of lightsaber MMA that offered Chris something he hadn't found elsewhere.

Training in lightsaber MMA became a transformative experience for Chris. The rhythmic movements and focused combat sequences provided a meditative outlet, helping to quiet the persistent noise of anxiety and stress that often accompanied PTSD. The physical exertion was therapeutic, not just in releasing tension but in fostering a sense of accomplishment and control – elements that are often challenging for those coping with PTSD.

But perhaps the most significant aspect of Chris's journey with lightsaber MMA was the sense of community and belonging he found. The lightsaber MMA community was inclusive and supportive, offering a space where Chris felt understood and accepted. This camaraderie was crucial in helping him open up and share his experiences, breaking the isolation that PTSD often brings.

Chris often shared how lightsaber MMA provided him with a new lens to view his challenges. The practice taught him to channel his energy positively, to focus on the present moment, and to build resilience not just physically but mentally and emotionally. It was a practice that combined the rigor of martial arts with the cathartic release of creative expression – a perfect blend for someone navigating the complex journey of healing from PTSD.

One particular moment stands out in Chris's journey. During a sparring session, amidst the intense focus and swift movements, Chris experienced a moment of profound clarity and peace. It was a realization that, within the controlled environment of lightsaber combat, he could confront his fears and anxieties in a way that was both empowering and healing. This moment was a turning point, marking a significant step in his journey towards managing his PTSD.

Chris's story is a powerful reminder of the healing potential of embracing new practices like lightsaber MMA. It underscores the fact that sometimes, the path to healing and coping with life's challenges can be found in the most unexpected places. Chris's journey with lightsaber MMA is not just about learning a new martial art; it's about the journey of reclaiming control, finding community, and rediscovering joy in life.

Brian's Story: Embracing Strength Through Lightsaber MMA

Let me share with you an inspiring story of transformation and empowerment – the story of Brian, a high-functioning individual on the autism spectrum, who found a new avenue of expression and coping through lightsaber MMA. Brian's journey is a powerful example of how embracing new challenges and engaging in innovative practices can lead to significant personal growth and improved well-being.

Brian had always found social interactions challenging and often felt overwhelmed in group settings. His world was a place of structure and routine, where predictability was a comfort. However, his passion for science fiction and his fascination with martial arts led him to discover a class on lightsaber MMA. This discovery marked the beginning of a transformative journey.

At first, Brian was hesitant to join the class, fearing the unpredictability and potential sensory overload. But the allure of the lightsaber, a symbol from the stories he cherished, drew him in. The first few sessions were challenging, but Brian's resilience shone through. He found the structured nature of the martial arts component of lightsaber MMA familiar and reassuring, and the creative aspect of lightsaber combat intriguing.

Training in lightsaber MMA offered Brian a unique blend of physical activity, mental engagement, and emotional expression. The physical routines helped in channeling his energy and reducing anxiety. The rhythmic movements and the focus required in lightsaber combat provided a meditative quality, helping Brian to center himself and manage sensory overstimulation.

One of the most significant aspects of Brian's journey was the improvement in his social interactions. The lightsaber MMA community was welcoming and inclusive, providing a safe and supportive environment where Brian could interact with others at his own pace. This interaction was not forced but evolved naturally through shared interests and mutual respect. Gradually, Brian found himself more comfortable in social settings, sharing his thoughts and even offering tips to fellow practitioners.

Brian's instructors played a crucial role in his journey. They were attuned to his needs, offering guidance and support while respecting his space and pace of learning. They celebrated his strengths and helped him navigate his challenges, fostering a sense of belonging and confidence in Brian.

Perhaps the most poignant moment in Brian's journey was during a group demonstration, where he showcased his lightsaber skills. The confidence and focus he displayed were a stark contrast to the shy individual who had first walked into the dojo. It was a moment of triumph, not just in mastering the lightsaber but in overcoming personal barriers.

Brian's story is a testament to the transformative power of embracing new and innovative practices like lightsaber MMA. It highlights the importance of inclusive communities and supportive environments in fostering growth and development, especially for individuals navigating the complexities of high-functioning autism. Brian's journey with lightsaber MMA is a reminder that within each of us lies untapped potential, and sometimes, all it takes is the right environment and a spark of interest to bring it to light.

3. Benefits: Physical, Mental, and Community Enhancement

In our pursuit of personal growth and self-improvement, it's essential to recognize how activities like lightsaber Mixed Martial Arts (MMA) can offer comprehensive benefits – physically, mentally, and within the community. Let's delve deeper into these aspects, understanding how each dimension contributes to our overall well-being and personal development.

Physical Benefits: A Holistic Approach to Fitness

The physical benefits of practicing lightsaber MMA are extensive and multifaceted. Unlike traditional martial arts, which may focus on specific aspects of physical training, lightsaber MMA offers a more holistic approach.

- Enhanced Cardiovascular Health:

The dynamic nature of lightsaber combat, with its fast-paced movements and intensive sparring sessions, significantly boosts cardiovascular endurance. Practitioners experience improvements in heart health and stamina, essential for overall physical well-being.

- Improved Strength and Flexibility:

Lightsaber MMA requires a unique combination of strength to wield the lightsaber effectively and flexibility to perform various combat moves. This combination leads to a more balanced physical conditioning, enhancing both power and agility.

• Coordination and Reflexes:

The practice demands a high level of coordination and quick reflexes. Regular training sharpens these skills, translating into improved performance in lightsaber MMA and other daily activities.

Mental Benefits: Beyond Physical Mastery

The mental benefits of lightsaber MMA are as significant as the physical ones. The discipline fosters a range of cognitive and emotional skills that contribute to mental health and resilience.

• Strategic Thinking and Problem-Solving:

Lightsaber combat is not just about physical prowess; it's about outsmarting your opponent. Practitioners develop enhanced strategic thinking and problem-solving skills as they learn to anticipate and counter their opponent's moves.

• Focus and Mindfulness:

The practice requires a high level of concentration, encouraging a state of mindfulness. This focus can help reduce stress and anxiety, promoting a sense of calm and mental clarity.

• Emotional Regulation:

Engaging in lightsaber MMA provides a healthy outlet for expressing emotions. The discipline required in training and the exhilaration of combat help in managing emotions, boosting confidence and fostering a positive self-image.

Community Benefits: Building Bonds and Fostering Inclusion

Perhaps one of the most significant aspects of lightsaber MMA is the community it builds. This martial art doesn't just create fighters; it fosters a sense of belonging and inclusion.

• Social Connection and Support:

The lightsaber MMA community is diverse and welcoming, allowing practitioners to connect with people from various backgrounds. These social connections offer support, encouragement, and a sense of belonging.

• Inclusivity and Diversity:

Lightsaber MMA attracts a wide range of individuals, making it a diverse and inclusive practice. This diversity enriches the training experience, as practitioners learn from each other's unique perspectives and experiences.

• Collective Growth and Learning:

Being part of the lightsaber MMA community means growing and learning together. The collaborative environment encourages sharing knowledge, experiences, and techniques, contributing to the collective growth of the group.

The practice of lightsaber MMA offers extensive benefits that encompass physical fitness, mental acuity, and community building. It's a discipline that not only trains the body but also nurtures the mind and soul. By engaging in lightsaber MMA, practitioners embark on a journey of comprehensive self-improvement, finding strength, resilience, and connection in the process.

The Transformation of Michael: Beyond Physical Fitness with Lightsaber Mixed Martial Arts

Let me share with you a truly inspiring story about Michael, someone I know whose experience with lightsaber MMA transcends physical fitness and touches the realms of mental resilience and community building. Michael's journey is a powerful illustration of how embracing innovative practices like lightsaber MMA can lead to transformative life changes, extending well beyond the confines of physical well-being.

Michael, a software engineer in his mid-thirties, always struggled with social anxiety and a sense of isolation. He found solace in his world of technology but longed for a connection that went beyond the digital realm. Michael's introduction to lightsaber MMA happened almost by chance when he saw a group practicing in a local park. Drawn by the energy and the unmistakable sound of lightsabers clashing, he decided to observe, his curiosity piqued.

What he saw was a revelation – a diverse group of individuals, all immersed in an activity that was both physically engaging and joyfully expressive. The following week, with some trepidation, Michael joined the group. The initial sessions were challenging, not just physically but also in terms of stepping into an unfamiliar social environment. However, the welcoming and supportive nature of the lightsaber MMA community began to ease his apprehension.

Over the weeks and months that followed, a remarkable transformation unfolded. Physically, Michael grew stronger and more agile, but the more significant changes were mental and emotional. The discipline required in lightsaber MMA, combined with constant strategic thinking and adaptability, sharpened his cognitive skills. He found himself more focused and mentally agile, not just during practice but in his professional life as well.

The most profound impact, however, was on Michael's social interactions. The lightsaber MMA community provided a space where he felt accepted and valued. It was a place where he could share his passion for science fiction and martial arts, forming connections that were rooted in shared interests and mutual respect. Gradually, his confidence in social settings began to grow. He started participating in group discussions, sharing tips with newer members, and even volunteering to help organize community events.

Michael often reflects on his journey with lightsaber MMA as a journey of self-discovery. He credits the practice with not only improving his physical fitness but also helping him overcome social barriers. He found a sense of belonging and a community that embraced him for who he was. The mental clarity and confidence he gained through lightsaber MMA extended into all areas of his life, enabling him to engage with the world in ways he never thought possible.

Michael's story is a testament to the transformative power of lightsaber MMA. It highlights how this innovative practice offers much more than physical training; it provides a pathway to mental resilience, emotional growth, and social connection. It's a reminder that sometimes, the key to unlocking our potential lies in stepping out of our comfort zones and embracing new experiences.

4. How to Begin Your Journey in Lightsaber MMA

Embarking on Your Lightsaber MMA Journey

Embarking on a journey in lightsaber Mixed Martial Arts (MMA) is a step towards not just learning a new martial art, but also discovering new facets of yourself. This journey is about embracing change, challenging your limits, and joining a community of like-minded enthusiasts. Let's explore the steps you can take to begin your transformative journey in lightsaber MMA.

- 1. Cultivate a Mindset of Exploration and Growth
  The first step in starting your lightsaber MMA journey is to cultivate the right mindset. Approach this new discipline with a sense of exploration and an eagerness to grow. Be open to new experiences and willing to step out of your comfort zone. Remember, every expert was once a beginner. Embrace the journey with the curiosity of a learner and the resilience of a warrior.

- 2. Research and Understand Lightsaber MMA
  Begin by immersing yourself in the world of lightsaber MMA. Research online, watch videos of practitioners and read about the discipline's techniques and philosophies. Understanding the history and principles of lightsaber MMA will give you a solid foundation and deepen your appreciation for this unique martial art. A good starting place is www.LightSwordMartialArts.com

- 3. Find the Right Training Facility or Instructor

Look for a dojo or training facility that offers lightsaber MMA classes. Ensure that the instructors are qualified and that the classes cater to different skill levels. It's important to find an environment where you feel comfortable and supported, one that aligns with your learning style and goals. Don't hesitate to visit multiple locations or talk to different instructors to find the right fit.

- 4. Equip Yourself Appropriately

While the most important aspect of lightsaber MMA is the skill and discipline, having the right equipment is also essential. Start with the basics – a practice lightsaber that's comfortable for you to handle. As you progress, you can invest in more advanced gear. Remember, the equipment should enhance your experience, not hinder it.

- 5. Start with the Basics and Be Patient

Lightsaber MMA, like any martial art, requires patience and persistence. Begin with the basics – understanding the stance, grip, and basic movements. Don't rush the process. Mastery comes with time and practice. Celebrate your progress, no matter how small, and be patient with yourself as you learn.

- 6. Engage with the Lightsaber MMA Community

One of the most enriching aspects of lightsaber MMA is its community. Engage with other practitioners, both in your dojo and online. Join forums, attend community events, and participate in group practice sessions. The lightsaber MMA community is a great source of support, learning, and inspiration. You can begin by visiting www.SaberNet.App

- 7. Set Goals and Track Your Progress
  Setting clear goals can help maintain your motivation and give direction to your training. Whether it's mastering a particular technique, participating in a sparring session, or simply improving your fitness, having goals keeps you focused. Regularly track your progress and celebrate your achievements along the way.

- 8. Stay Open to Continuous Learning
  Finally, remember that the journey in lightsaber MMA is one of continuous learning. There's always something new to discover, be it a technique, a strategy, or a facet of your personality. Stay open and committed to lifelong learning, and embrace each step of your journey with enthusiasm and dedication.

Embarking on your lightsaber MMA journey is not just about physical training; it's about embarking on a journey of self-discovery and personal growth. It's about finding a balance between discipline and creativity, strength and agility, individual achievement, and community spirit. So, take that first step with confidence, and embrace the incredible journey that awaits you in the world of lightsaber MMA.

* * *

Footnotes

Holistic Benefits of Martial Arts: A systematic review of hard martial arts in adults shows that the majority of studies reported positive effects resulting from hard martial arts practice, indicating improvements and maintenance in balance, cognitive function, and psychological health. These benefits are attainable regardless of the age at which practice is commenced◇0†source◇◇146†source◇.

Psychological Impacts of Combat Sports: It has been theorized that martial arts reduce aggressive tendencies by enabling participants to channel such energies into productive and self-enhancing activities. The development of self-control and enhanced awareness of self-boundaries are also thought to contribute to this observed psychological benefits◇148†source◇1. Additionally, limited research suggests martial arts training may be an efficacious sports-based mental health intervention, potentially providing an inexpensive alternative to psychological therapy1. Martial arts training has been shown to have a significant but small positive effect on well-being and a medium effect on internalizing mental health outcomes1.

Integrating Traditional and Modern Martial Arts Practices: The integration of martial arts practices like Tai Chi and Qi Gong into Western medical practices is a time-honored tradition with a growing body of research affirming the health benefits of these ancient arts. These practices, known for balancing the body's nervous system and enhancing overall health and vitality, offer unique advantages from improving physical strength and agility to fostering mental clarity and emotional equilibrium◇175†source◇. They are recognized for their therapeutic potential in Western culture, especially in high-stress environments, and are increasingly being integrated into rehabilitation programs for their non-pharmacological benefits in managing conditions like chronic pain1. The growing adoption of martial arts practices in Western healthcare settings reflects a return to holistic health principles, highlighting these ancient methods as effective tools for modern healing◇177†source◇.

These references underscore the comprehensive benefits of martial arts, illustrating how they extend beyond physical fitness to encompass mental and emotional well-being, and how the fusion of traditional and modern practices is gaining recognition and validity in various health and wellness spheres.

CHAPTER THREE

Debunking Traditional Martial Arts Myths

Challenging Outdated Martial Arts Beliefs
- Defining common misconceptions
- Stories debunking traditional martial arts myths
- Beyond Physical Prowess: The Mental Game
- The Diversity and Adaptability of Modern Martial Arts
- The Practicality of Lightsaber MMA in Real-World Scenarios

Subsection: Challenging Outdated Martial Arts Beliefs

*1. Defining Common Misconceptions:
Unraveling the Misconceptions*

In this journey of martial arts enlightenment, it's pivotal to unravel the misconceptions shrouding traditional martial arts. These misconceptions, like invisible chains, often limit our exploration and growth in the vast and dynamic world of martial arts.

- **Rethinking Fixed Abilities**: The belief that our martial arts abilities are static is a misconception we must overcome. Growth and adaptability are at the heart of martial arts. Embrace the idea that with dedication and the right strategies, your martial arts prowess can evolve beyond current limitations.

- **Reframing Fear**: Often, fear is mistakenly perceived as a signal to retreat. Instead, let's view fear as a catalyst for growth, pushing us toward uncharted territories in martial arts where true learning happens. Fear indicates areas ripe for development and mastery.

- **Redefining Failure**: Instead of viewing failure as a defeat, let's redefine it as an opportunity for learning. Each misstep in martial arts is a chance to gain insights and come back stronger. The path to mastery is paved with lessons learned from failures.

- **Success as a Journey**: Success in martial arts is not a final destination but an ongoing journey. It's about continual improvement and adaptation, not just reaching a set goal. Focus on evolving your skills and techniques, and success will become a byproduct of this lifelong journey.

- **Embracing Change**: The misconception that change is too difficult limits growth in martial arts. Change is not just possible; it's necessary. Start with small, consistent steps, and soon, you'll find yourself achieving transformations that once seemed insurmountable.

By challenging these outdated beliefs and misconceptions, we open ourselves to a richer, more fulfilling martial arts experience. It's about breaking free from the confines of traditional thinking and embracing a more dynamic and adaptable approach to martial arts. Remember, the only limits that exist are the ones we place on ourselves. Let's break these barriers and step into a world of unlimited martial arts potential.

2. Stories debunking traditional martial arts myths

"Debunking the Idea that Traditional Martial Arts are the Only Authentic Form of Combat Training"

In the dynamic world of combat training, there's a prevalent idea that only traditional martial arts represent the authentic form of combat training. This notion, deeply rooted in respect for ancient practices, often overlooks the evolving nature of martial arts and combat needs in our modern world. Let's dive into debunking this idea, embracing a more inclusive and progressive perspective.

1. **Understanding the Evolution of Combat Training**: Combat training, like any discipline, evolves. Traditional martial arts have laid a solid foundation, emphasizing discipline, technique, and mental conditioning. However, the world we live in today is vastly different from when these arts were developed. Our understanding of the human body, psychology, and combat tactics has grown. To stay relevant and effective, combat training must evolve, integrating new insights and techniques. This evolution doesn't diminish the value of traditional martial arts; it enhances and complements them.

2. **Recognizing the Diversity in Combat Needs**: Today's combat scenarios – be they for self-defense, sport, or professional training – are diverse and complex. Relying solely on traditional methods may limit one's ability to adapt to varied situations. Modern combat training, which often integrates various martial arts styles and contemporary techniques, offers a more versatile skill set that's crucial for today's diverse combat needs.

3. **Embracing Innovation and Adaptability**: Innovation is key in any field, and combat training is no exception. Practices like Mixed Martial Arts (MMA) demonstrate the effectiveness of combining different martial arts styles. These innovative approaches offer a more holistic training experience, covering a wider range of techniques and strategies. Adaptability, a critical skill in combat, is best developed through exposure to various styles and scenarios – something that modern, integrated training approaches excel at.

4. **Respecting Tradition While Encouraging Growth**: Debunking this idea isn't about disrespecting traditional martial arts – it's about acknowledging that growth and improvement are always possible. We can honor and preserve the rich heritage of traditional martial arts while also recognizing the benefits of modern approaches. It's about finding a balance between tradition and innovation.

5. **The Role of Personal Goals and Preferences**: Ultimately, the choice of combat training depends on personal goals and preferences. Some may find fulfillment in the structure and heritage of traditional martial arts, while others may seek the dynamism and diversity of modern styles. Both paths are valid and authentic in their own right.

6. **Encouraging an Open-Minded Approach**: As we continue to grow and learn in our combat training journeys, let's encourage

an open-minded approach. Explore different styles, learn from various disciplines, and find what works best for you. The authenticity of combat training lies not in its adherence to tradition, but in its effectiveness, adaptability, and ability to grow with its practitioners.

The idea that traditional martial arts are the only authentic form of combat training is a limited perspective. By embracing both traditional and modern approaches, we can benefit from a more comprehensive and adaptable combat training experience, suited to the complexities of our modern world. Remember, the journey of combat training is as diverse as the individuals who embark on it – there's no one-size-fits-all approach. Embrace diversity, encourage innovation, and stay open to the vast possibilities that the world of combat training offers.

"Real-life examples where Lightsaber MMA has provided effective and practical combat skills."

In the world of martial arts, the emergence of Lightsaber MMA has been a game-changer, blending the time-honored traditions of classic martial arts with the innovative and dynamic aspects of lightsaber combat. Let's explore some real-life examples that highlight the effectiveness and practicality of the combat skills honed through Lightsaber MMA training.

Self-Defense Situations:
James, a Lightsaber MMA enthusiast, shared how his training helped him during a precarious situation. Walking home late one night, he found himself confronted by an aggressor. James's Lightsaber MMA training kicked in, enabling him to defuse the situation with confidence and control, using defensive maneuvers he had practiced in class. His ability to stay calm, assess the situation, and react appropriately was a

direct result of his Lightsaber MMA training.

Professional Security Personnel:
Lisa, who works in private security, incorporated Lightsaber MMA into her regular training regimen. She found that the unique blend of traditional martial arts techniques with the agility and reflex training from lightsaber combat greatly enhanced her capabilities. In various real-life scenarios, Lisa used the skills she developed in Lightsaber MMA – from maintaining situational awareness to handling physical confrontations – demonstrating the practical application of these skills in her profession.

Improving Athletic Performance in Other Sports:
Nick, a competitive athlete in another sport, took up Lightsaber MMA as cross-training. He noticed significant improvements in his primary sport, attributing these to the enhanced reflexes, agility, and strategic thinking developed through Lightsaber MMA. This cross-training approach helped him anticipate his opponents' moves better and react more quickly, giving him a competitive edge.

Empowering the Youth:
A youth coach, Sam, integrated Lightsaber MMA into her program for at-risk teens. She observed remarkable changes in her students, who not only learned practical self-defense skills but also developed greater self-discipline, focus, and confidence. The program's success in positively impacting these young lives showcased Lightsaber MMA's practicality beyond physical combat skills, extending into life skills and personal development.

Building Confidence in Everyday Life:
Ben, initially a shy and introverted individual, found that training in Lightsaber MMA significantly boosted his confidence and social skills. The training sessions, which required interaction and cooperation with fellow practitioners, helped him open up and connect with others, skills

he later transferred to his personal and professional life.

These real-life examples illustrate the broad spectrum of practical benefits offered by Lightsaber MMA. From enhancing self-defense capabilities to improving professional competencies, and from aiding personal development to fostering social connections, Lightsaber MMA offers a holistic approach to combat training. It stands as a testament to the idea that martial arts training can be both practical and transformative, equipping individuals with skills that extend far beyond the dojo.

"Benefits of Integrating Modern Techniques like Lightsaber MMA into Martial Arts Training"

In our pursuit of excellence, it's essential to recognize the power of integrating modern techniques like Lightsaber MMA into martial arts training. This blend of traditional discipline with innovative practices offers a multitude of benefits, creating a comprehensive approach to self-improvement. Let's explore these benefits in depth.

Enhanced Physical Conditioning:

Lightsaber MMA combines the precision and discipline of traditional martial arts with the dynamic, high-energy movements of modern combat techniques. This fusion results in enhanced physical conditioning. You're not just training for strength or agility; you're developing a well-rounded physical fitness that prepares you for various challenges, both in and out of the dojo.

Mental and Cognitive Advancements:

The strategic nature of Lightsaber MMA sharpens your mental faculties. It demands quick thinking, adaptability, and decision-making under pressure. These skills, honed through practice, translate into improved cognitive abilities in everyday life. Imagine facing life's challenges with the same strategic approach and mental agility you use in Lightsaber MMA training.

Increased Engagement and Motivation:

Let's face it, traditional martial arts can sometimes feel repetitive. The introduction of Lightsaber MMA adds a new level of excitement and engagement. This modern twist keeps training fresh and motivating, inspiring you to consistently show up and put in your best effort.

Building Confidence and Self-Esteem:

Mastering the techniques of Lightsaber MMA is empowering. There's a unique confidence that comes from wielding a lightsaber with skill and precision. This confidence spills over into other areas of your life, enhancing your self-esteem and overall self-image.

Fostering Creativity and Self-Expression:

Lightsaber MMA encourages creativity. It's not just about following set patterns; it's about expressing yourself through movement. This creative aspect of training allows you to explore and develop your unique style, fostering a sense of individuality and self-expression.

Promoting Inclusivity and Community:

The world of Lightsaber MMA is diverse and inclusive. It attracts people from various backgrounds, each bringing their unique perspective. This diversity enriches the training environment, fostering a sense of community and belonging. In the dojo, we're all on the same journey of growth and discovery, supporting and learning from one another.

Adapting to Modern Self-Defense Needs:

The techniques and strategies learned in Lightsaber MMA are practical and applicable to modern self-defense scenarios. They teach you to assess situations quickly, respond effectively, and protect yourself in a variety of contexts.

Lifelong Learning and Adaptability:
Integrating modern techniques like Lightsaber MMA into martial arts training embodies the principle of lifelong learning. It's about staying adaptable, open to new ideas, and continuously evolving your skills. In a world that's constantly changing, this adaptability is key to both personal and professional success.

Incorporating modern techniques like Lightsaber MMA into traditional martial arts training offers a balanced approach to personal development. It's about blending the best of both worlds – the discipline and wisdom of traditional martial arts with the innovation and excitement of modern practices. Embrace this fusion, and you'll find yourself not just a better martial artist, but a more rounded, confident, and adaptable individual, ready to take on whatever challenges life throws your way.

Opening Your Mind to New Forms of Martial Arts: Exploring Lightsaber MMA

In our journey toward growth and self-discovery, it's vital to open our minds to new possibilities and experiences. Today, I want to talk about embracing new forms of martial arts, specifically Lightsaber MMA, and how this innovative practice can enrich your life.

First, let's address a common mindset – the hesitation to try something new, especially when it challenges traditional beliefs. It's natural to feel a sense of loyalty to the familiar but remember, growth often happens outside our comfort zones. Lightsaber MMA, a blend of traditional martial arts techniques with the dynamic and imaginative aspects of lightsaber combat, offers a unique opportunity for physical, mental, and emotional growth.

Physical Benefits: A New Challenge

Engaging in Lightsaber MMA presents a new physical challenge. It combines the discipline and precision of traditional martial arts with the agility and creativity of lightsaber handling. This fusion not only enhances your physical fitness but also adds an element of fun and excitement to your workout routine. It pushes your body in new ways, helping you discover strengths you might not have known you had.

Mental Benefits: Strategic Thinking and Focus

Lightsaber MMA is not just about physical prowess; it's about strategy and mental agility. Each movement, each combat sequence, requires focus, quick thinking, and adaptability. This practice sharpens your mind, enhances your problem-solving skills, and improves your ability to concentrate under pressure – skills that are invaluable in all areas of life.

Emotional Benefits: Confidence and Expression

This innovative form of martial arts is a powerful tool for building confidence and self-expression. The act of wielding a lightsaber, mastering its movements, and engaging in combat can be incredibly empowering. It provides an outlet for expressing yourself, for channeling your emotions into something constructive and creative.

Community and Connection

One of the most beautiful aspects of Lightsaber MMA is the community it builds. This inclusive and diverse community brings together people from all walks of life, united by a shared passion. It's a space where you can form meaningful connections, learn from others, and be part of a supportive and motivating environment.

Opening Your Mind to New Experiences

So, how can you open your mind to this new form of martial arts? Start by researching Lightsaber MMA – watch videos, read articles, and maybe attend a class or a demonstration. Talk to practitioners, learn from their experiences, and see firsthand the joy and fulfillment they derive from this practice.

Taking the First Step

If you feel drawn to Lightsaber MMA, take that first step. Sign up for a class, engage with the community, and permit yourself to be a beginner. Remember, every master was once a novice. Be patient with yourself, enjoy the learning process, and celebrate each milestone on this journey.

Embracing Lifelong Learning

Finally, embrace the mindset of lifelong learning. Whether it's Lightsaber MMA or any other new form of martial arts, the key is to remain open, curious, and eager to grow. These experiences enrich our lives, not just by teaching us new skills but by broadening our perspectives and connecting us with others.

Opening your mind to new forms of martial arts, like Lightsaber MMA, is a journey that offers rich rewards. It's an opportunity for physical, mental, and emotional growth, building confidence, fostering creativity, and connecting with a vibrant community. So, I encourage you to explore, step outside your comfort zone, and discover the limitless potential that lies within you. Remember, the only limit to your impact is your imagination and commitment.

3. Beyond Physical Prowess: The Mental Game

Another myth is that martial arts are all about physical strength. Let's shift that perspective! Lightsaber MMA places equal emphasis on mental strategy and emotional control – elements crucial in modern combat scenarios.

"Challenging the Notion that Physical Strength is the Sole Focus of Martial Arts"

In the realm of martial arts, there's a prevailing notion that physical strength is the primary focus. However, this perspective is limited and overlooks the multifaceted essence of martial arts. Let's challenge this notion and explore how martial arts' training is about so much more than just physical prowess.

Mental and Emotional Strength:
Martial arts' training is as much a mental and emotional journey as it is a physical one. It teaches discipline, focus, and resilience. Practitioners learn to control their minds, manage emotions, and develop a mental toughness that is invaluable in all aspects of life. The patience and per-severance developed in mastering martial arts techniques translate into strong mental fortitude.

Strategic Thinking and Problem Solving:
Martial arts require strategic thinking and quick decision-making skills. It's about anticipating your opponent's moves, understanding their strategy, and adapting your own. This aspect of martial arts hones cognitive abilities, making you not just a stronger person physically, but also a more adept and strategic thinker.

Spiritual Growth and Self-Discovery:
Many martial arts disciplines incorporate a significant spiritual element. Training often involves meditation, reflection, and a journey of self-discovery. Practitioners learn about themselves at a deeper level, gaining insights into their character, strengths, and areas for growth.

Community and Relationships:
The martial arts community is a vital part of the training experience. It's about building relationships, learning from others, and growing together. This sense of community fosters social skills, empathy, and a sense of belonging, which are crucial for our emotional well-being.

Health and Wellness Beyond Strength:
While physical strength is a component of martial arts, the benefits extend to overall health and wellness. Regular practice improves cardiovascular health, flexibility, balance, and coordination. It's a holistic approach to fitness that benefits the entire body and mind.

Empowerment and Confidence:
Training in martial arts empowers individuals. It builds confidence not just in one's physical abilities but also in their capacity to face challenges, overcome obstacles, and stands up for themselves and others. This empowerment extends beyond the dojo into everyday life.

Adaptability and Resilience:
Martial arts teach adaptability and resilience. You learn to be flexible, to adjust to new challenges, and to bounce back from setbacks. These skills are essential in a world that is constantly changing and evolving.

Challenging the notion that martial arts are solely about physical strength opens our eyes to the rich, multidimensional nature of this discipline. It's a holistic practice that develops the body, sharpens the mind, nurtures the spirit, and strengthens emotional resilience. As we embrace this broader understanding of martial arts, we empower our-selves to grow in every aspect of our lives, becoming not just physically strong but well-rounded, resilient, and empowered individuals.

The Mental and Strategic Depth in Lightsaber MMA: Inspiring Stories

Let me share with you the captivating stories of individuals who discovered the profound mental and strategic depth offered by Light-saber MMA. These stories not only demonstrate the physical prowess required but also illuminate the mental and emotional growth fostered through this modern martial art.

Elena's Journey to Mental Clarity:
Elena, a graphic designer, turned to Lightsaber MMA during a period of intense career stress. She found that the focus required in mastering lightsaber techniques helped clear her mind. The strategic thinking involved in lightsaber combat, where anticipating an oppo-nent's move is key, mirrored the problem-solving skills she needed in her job. Elena credits Lightsaber MMA with enhancing her mental clarity and strategic thinking, enabling her to approach her career challenges with a fresh perspective.

Marcus's Path to Emotional Resilience:
Marcus, a former soldier, struggled with emotional regulation fol-lowing his service. He discovered Lightsaber MMA and found in it a discipline that challenged him both physically and mentally. The intense focus and mental discipline required in lightsaber combat provided him with a way to channel his emotions positively. Gradually, he developed greater emotional resilience and a sense of inner peace. Marcus's story is a testament to the power of martial arts in providing mental balance

and emotional strength.

Sophia's Tactical Mastery:

As a competitive player in strategic games, Sophia was drawn to Lightsaber MMA for its combination of physical engagement and mental strategy. She found that the tactics and quick decision-making required in Lightsaber MMA improved her analytical skills. Training sessions became her playground for testing strategies, improving her reaction time, and sharpening her tactical mind. Sophia's experience highlights how Lightsaber MMA enhances cognitive abilities, making it a perfect blend of physical and mental exercise.

Tony's Community-driven Growth:

Tony, initially introverted and socially anxious, joined a Lightsaber MMA club seeking a new hobby. He found a supportive community where strategic discussions about combat techniques and mental preparation were commonplace. Engaging with others in strategizing and planning combat sequences helped Tony develop his communication skills and boosted his confidence. This social aspect of Lightsaber MMA, where sharing knowledge and strategies is encouraged, played a crucial role in Tony's mental and emotional growth.

These stories demonstrate that Lightsaber MMA is more than just a physical activity; it's a mental and strategic discipline that fosters cognitive development, emotional resilience, and social skills. The strategic depth of Lightsaber MMA is evident in the way it transforms individuals, not just in their physical abilities but in their mental and emotional capacities as well. Remember, the journey in martial arts, including Lightsaber MMA, is not just about the body. It's about the mind, the heart, and the spirit coming together in a dance of discipline, strategy, and growth.

"Benefits of a Balanced Approach to Mental and Physical Training in Lightsaber MMA"

In the quest for personal development and mastery, a balanced approach to both mental and physical training in Lightsaber Mixed Martial Arts (MMA) is crucial. This unique martial art form isn't just about the physical prowess of wielding a lightsaber; it's equally about mental fortitude and strategic thinking. Let's delve into the benefits of this balanced approach.

Enhanced Physical Fitness:
Lightsaber MMA provides a comprehensive physical workout that improves strength, agility, and flexibility. This training goes beyond traditional exercises, incorporating dynamic movements that challenge the body in new and exciting ways. It's about building a body that is not only strong but also adaptable and resilient.

Cognitive Development:
The strategic aspects of Lightsaber MMA hone cognitive abilities. It requires practitioners to think on their feet, anticipate opponents' moves, and make quick decisions. This mental engagement sharpens the mind, enhances problem-solving skills, and boosts decision-making abilities, translating into improved cognitive functions in everyday life.

Emotional Regulation and Resilience:
Engaging in Lightsaber MMA is also an emotional journey. The discipline required in training, the thrill of combat, and the satisfaction of mastering new skills contributes to emotional growth. Practitioners learn to manage stress, control their emotions, and develop resilience – qualities that are invaluable in all aspects of life.

Mind-Body Connection:
A key benefit of a balanced Lightsaber MMA training regimen is the development of a strong mind-body connection. This training

promotes mindfulness, where practitioners are fully present at the moment, aware of their movements, and in tune with their bodies. This mindfulness enhances overall well-being and brings a sense of inner peace.

Strategic Thinking and Planning:
Lightsaber MMA is not just about physical combat; it's a game of strategy. Practitioners learn to analyze situations, plan their moves, and adapt their strategies on the go. This strategic thinking is a powerful skill, applicable in personal and professional life, where strategic planning and adaptability are keys to success.

Building Confidence and Self-Esteem:
Mastering the techniques of Lightsaber MMA builds confidence. There's a sense of achievement and empowerment in learning to handle a lightsaber with skill and precision. This confidence extends beyond the dojo, enhancing self-esteem and self-belief in various life situations.

Social Skills and Community Building:
Lightsaber MMA training is often conducted in groups, providing an opportunity to build social skills and be part of a community. Practitioners learn to communicate, work as a team, and support each other, fostering a sense of belonging and community spirit.

A balanced approach to mental and physical training in Lightsaber MMA offers a plethora of benefits. It's a holistic development journey that enhances physical fitness, sharpens the mind, nurtures emotional well-being, and fosters social connections. By embracing this balanced approach, practitioners of Lightsaber MMA can achieve a harmonious development of body, mind, and spirit, equipping them with the skills and confidence to succeed in all areas of life.

"Incorporating Mental Training Exercises into Your Martial Arts Routine: Enhancing Lightsaber MMA Training"

Incorporating mental training exercises into your martial arts routine can elevate your practice to new heights. Let's explore some examples of mental training exercises that can be seamlessly integrated into your Lightsaber MMA training sessions.

Visualization Techniques:

Before beginning your training session, take a moment to visualize your movements. Close your eyes and imagine yourself executing perfect strikes, blocks, and maneuvers with your lightsaber. Visualization is a powerful tool that enhances muscle memory and prepares your mind for physical action.

Mindful Breathing Exercises:

Incorporate mindful breathing exercises into your warm-up routine. Concentrate on deep, rhythmic breaths to center your mind and bring focus to the present moment. This practice not only calms your mind but also optimizes your body's oxygen flow, enhancing your performance during training.

Strategic Planning Drills:

During sparring sessions, take brief pauses to reflect and plan your next moves. This exercise develops your strategic thinking, helping you to anticipate your opponent's moves and respond effectively. It's about being two steps ahead in your mind.

Stress Management Techniques:

After intense training or sparring, practice stress management techniques like progressive muscle relaxation or guided meditation. This helps in releasing any built-up tension and trains you to maintain composure and calmness, essential traits in martial arts.

Emotional Regulation Training:

Engage in scenarios that challenge your emotional responses. For instance, practice maintaining focus under deliberately distracting conditions. This strengthens your ability to control emotions like frustration or anger, which are crucial in high-stakes combat situations.

Cognitive Flexibility Exercises:

Include exercises that require quick decision-making and adaptability. Change up your routines frequently or practice reacting to unexpected scenarios during training. This enhances your cognitive flexibility, making you a more adaptable and versatile martial artist.

Concentration Drills:

Perform exercises that require high levels of concentration, such as practicing complex lightsaber forms or balancing drills. These activities improve your focus and attention span, crucial for mastering the art of Lightsaber MMA.

Positive Affirmation Practice:

Start and end your training sessions with positive affirmations. Remind yourself of your strengths, your progress, and your goals. This boosts your self-confidence and keeps you motivated.

Goal-Setting Sessions:

Regularly set and review your training goals. This practice not only keeps you aligned with your objectives but also train your mind to stay committed and driven.

Reflection and Journaling:

After training, spend time reflecting on your performance. Journal your thoughts, experiences, and areas for improvement. This reflective practice enhances self-awareness and aids in your martial arts journey.

Incorporating these mental training exercises into your Lightsaber MMA routine will lead to a more holistic development as a martial artist. It's about balancing the physical with the mental, the action with the strategy, and the strength with the resilience. Embrace these practices, and watch as they transform not just your martial arts skills, but also your approach to life's challenges. Remember, the greatest battles are often fought and won in the mind.

4. *The Diversity and Adaptability of Modern Martial Arts*

Some say traditional martial arts are the most adaptable and diverse – but is that the full picture? Lightsaber MMA proves otherwise with its inclusivity and flexibility, catering to a wide range of practitioners.

"Addressing the Misconception About the Lack of Diversity in Modern Martial Arts Like Lightsaber MMA"

In the dynamic world of martial arts, there's a prevalent misconception about the lack of diversity, particularly in modern forms like Lightsaber MMA. This view often stems from traditional images of martial arts and doesn't reflect the inclusive reality of these contemporary practices. Let's address and debunk this misconception.

Embracing a Wide Range of Practitioners:
Modern martial arts, including Lightsaber MMA, attract individuals from diverse backgrounds. These disciplines are no longer limited to a

specific age group, gender, or cultural background. In my own experience, I've seen people of all ages, professions, and walks of life engaging in Lightsaber MMA. It's a unifying practice that transcends traditional barriers, bringing together a rich tapestry of individuals, each contributing their unique perspective and experience.

Cultural Integration and Adaptation:

Lightsaber MMA, inspired by the iconic Star Wars saga, draws from a variety of cultural influences. This modern martial art form is not bound by the cultural and geographic origins that characterize traditional martial arts. Instead, it represents a blend of global influences, appealing to a broad, culturally diverse audience.

Promoting Inclusivity and Acceptance:

The community around modern martial arts like Lightsaber MMA is known for its inclusivity. These arts promote values of acceptance and respect, creating a welcoming environment for everyone. Practitioners learn not only martial arts skills but also the importance of empathy and understanding diverse perspectives.

Breaking Gender Stereotypes:

Another significant aspect of modern martial arts is their role in breaking gender stereotypes. Lightsaber MMA, for example, has a substantial number of female practitioners, who find empowerment and strength in this art form. It challenges the traditional notion that martial arts are predominantly male activities.

Adaptive Practices for Varied Abilities:

Modern martial arts are also adaptable, catering to people with different physical abilities. Lightsaber MMA can be modified to suit various fitness levels and physical conditions, making it accessible to a wider range of individuals. This adaptability is key to its growing popularity and diverse participation.

A Platform for Personal Expression:
Unlike traditional martial arts, which often emphasize conformity and adherence to set patterns, modern forms like Lightsaber MMA offer more room for personal expression. This aspect attracts people with varied interests and backgrounds, providing a creative outlet for self-expression through martial arts.

The misconception about the lack of diversity in modern martial arts like Lightsaber MMA is far from reality. These contemporary practices are at the forefront of promoting diversity, inclusivity, and cultural integration. By embracing and celebrating this diversity, we enrich our experiences and learnings in the martial arts world, making it a more vibrant and inclusive community. The true spirit of martial arts lies in its ability to unite, empower, and inspire people from all walks of life.

"Lightsaber MMA's Adaptability to Different Age Groups, Skill Levels, and Physical Abilities"

Lightsaber Mixed Martial Arts (MMA) stands out as a highly adaptable and inclusive discipline, catering to various age groups, skill levels, and physical abilities. Let me share some compelling examples illustrating this adaptability.

Youth Engagement:
In Lightsaber MMA, younger enthusiasts find a perfect blend of imaginative play and physical activity. It's tailored to be safe and fun, encouraging kids to develop coordination, discipline, and teamwork. For teenagers, it offers a unique way to channel energy positively while learning valuable life skills.

Adults and Skill Development:
Adults, irrespective of their initial skill level, find Lightsaber MMA both challenging and rewarding. Beginners start with basic techniques,

gradually advancing to more complex forms and sparring, ensuring steady progress. For experienced martial artists, Lightsaber MMA provides an opportunity to refine their skills and explore new combat strategies, keeping their practice dynamic and engaging.

Seniors and Gentle Practice:

Lightsaber MMA isn't just for the young or the highly skilled; it's also adaptable for seniors seeking an engaging way to stay active. Training can be modified to focus on gentle movements, balance, and flexibility, offering a low-impact form of exercise that is both enjoyable and beneficial for maintaining physical health.

Adaptations for Physical Disabilities:

The inclusivity of Lightsaber MMA extends to those with physical disabilities. Training programs can be adapted to meet individual needs, ensuring everyone has the opportunity to participate and benefit from the discipline. This adaptability fosters a sense of empowerment and belonging among all practitioners.

Therapeutic and Rehabilitative Aspects:

Lightsaber MMA can also be therapeutic. For individuals recovering from injuries or dealing with chronic conditions, it offers a form of rehabilitative exercise that can be tailored to their recovery process. This aspect of training aids in building strength, improving mobility, and enhancing overall well-being.

These examples demonstrate the remarkable versatility of Lightsaber MMA. It's a discipline that embraces diversity, offering a welcoming and inclusive environment for people from all walks of life. This adaptability is key to its growing popularity and its ability to provide a fulfilling experience to a wide range of practitioners.

"Highlighting the Inclusive Nature of Lightsaber MMA"

In the world of martial arts, Lightsaber MMA stands as a beacon of inclusivity, a discipline that opens its doors wide to everyone, irrespective of age, background, or physical capability. This modern form of martial arts, inspired by the legendary Star Wars saga, transcends traditional boundaries, creating a space where diversity is not just accepted but celebrated.

Welcoming All Ages:

One of the most striking aspects of Lightsaber MMA is its appeal across different age groups. For children, it's a gateway to learning discipline, focus, and respect, all wrapped in the excitement of wielding a lightsaber. For adults, it's an opportunity to engage in a physically and mentally stimulating activity that breaks the monotony of routine exercise. Even seniors find joy and a sense of community in Lightsaber MMA, proving that it's never too late to start a new journey in martial arts.

Adaptable to Various Skill Levels:

Whether you're a beginner with no prior experience in martial arts or a seasoned practitioner, Lightsaber MMA offers something for everyone. Instructors tailor training to individual skill levels, ensuring that each person is challenged yet not overwhelmed. This adaptability makes Lightsaber MMA a practice where everyone can grow at their own pace, without feeling left behind.

Inclusive of All Physical Abilities:

Recognizing that physical abilities vary widely, Lightsaber MMA prides itself on being accessible to people with different physical capabilities. Adaptive training methods are employed to ensure that everyone, including those with physical disabilities, can participate and benefit from the practice. This inclusiveness not only enriches the experience of all involved but also fosters a deeper understanding and appreciation for diversity.

A Melting Pot of Backgrounds and Cultures:

The global appeal of Star Wars translates into Lightsaber MMA, attracting enthusiasts from varied backgrounds and cultures. This melting pot creates a rich and dynamic environment where cultural exchanges are as common as lightsaber duels. Such diversity enhances the learning experience, as practitioners are exposed to different perspectives and ways of thinking.

Promoting Gender Equality:

Lightsaber MMA is a discipline where gender stereotypes are shattered. Men and women train together, learning from and supporting each other. This gender-inclusive environment empowers individuals, particularly women and girls, to discover their strength and assert their place not just in martial arts but in all areas of life.

Fostering a Sense of Belonging:

At the heart of Lightsaber MMA's inclusivity is the sense of community it builds. Here, you're not just a practitioner; you're part of a family that shares your passions and supports your growth. This sense of belonging is what makes Lightsaber MMA more than just a martial art; it's a movement that brings people together, united in their love for the discipline.

Lightsaber MMA is more than a physical or mental discipline; it's a testament to the power of inclusivity in martial arts. Welcoming people from all walks of life not only enriches the practice but also creates a community where everyone can thrive. As we embrace the inclusive nature of Lightsaber MMA, we learn that the true strength of martial arts lies in its ability to unite us in our diversity.

"Engaging with Diverse Martial Arts Communities and Trying Different Styles, Including Lightsaber MMA"

In the journey of self-improvement and discovery, one of the most exhilarating adventures is to engage with diverse martial arts communities and explore various styles, including the dynamic world of Lightsaber MMA. This exploration is not just about physical training; it's an expedition into diverse cultures, philosophies, and techniques that enrich our lives in profound ways.

The Value of Diverse Martial Arts Styles:
Every martial art style offers unique insights and techniques. From the disciplined precision of Karate to the fluid movements of Capoeira, each style embodies a different set of values and skills. Engaging with various martial arts communities exposes you to these differences, broadening your perspective and enhancing your overall martial arts proficiency.

Lightsaber MMA: A Fusion of Tradition and Innovation:
Lightsaber MMA stands out as a modern martial art that combines traditional martial arts principles with the imaginative and engaging aspects of lightsaber combat. It's a style that appeals to a broad audience, from Star Wars enthusiasts to serious martial artists and offers an exciting and inclusive environment for learning and growth.

Cultural Exchange and Understanding:
As you explore different martial arts communities, you immerse yourself in diverse cultural backgrounds. This cultural exchange fosters a deeper understanding and respect for people from different walks of life. It's a powerful way to build empathy and connect with others on a profound level.

Personal Growth and Flexibility:

Trying different martial arts styles, including Lightsaber MMA, challenges you to step out of your comfort zone. It tests your adaptability and willingness to learn, qualities that are essential for personal growth. Each style will challenge you in different ways, pushing you to grow not just physically but mentally and emotionally as well.

Building a Supportive Network:

Engaging with various martial arts communities allows you to build a network of support and friendship. These communities are often tight-knit groups that share a common passion for martial arts. They provide a support system that can motivate and inspire you to push beyond your limits.

Enhancing Physical and Mental Fitness:

Each martial arts style offers a unique approach to physical fitness and mental conditioning. By training in different styles, including Lightsaber MMA, you develop a more comprehensive fitness regimen that targets various aspects of your physical and mental health.

The Joy of Continuous Learning:

Martial arts are a lifelong journey of learning. Engaging with different styles keeps this journey exciting and fulfilling. There's always something new to learn, whether it's a new technique in Lightsaber MMA or a philosophical insight from Aikido.

Engaging with diverse martial arts communities and trying different styles, including Lightsaber MMA, is a journey that offers immense rewards. It enriches your martial arts practice, opens your mind to new perspectives, and connects you with a diverse network of practitioners. This journey is a testament to the unifying power of martial arts and its ability to inspire personal growth and understanding across different cultures and communities. In the world of martial arts, the greatest strength lies in the diversity of its many styles.

5. The Practicality of Lightsaber MMA in Real-World Scenarios

A common misconception is that Lightsaber MMA isn't practical for real-world defense. However, its principles are deeply rooted in practicality, blending traditional defense techniques with modern, realistic applications.

"Debunking Myths About the Impracticality of Lightsaber MMA"

There's a common myth that Lightsaber Mixed Martial Arts (MMA) is impractical, viewed by some as mere fantasy play rather than a legitimate form of martial arts. Today, let's debunk this misconception and illuminate the practical and substantial benefits of Lightsaber MMA.

Physical Fitness and Coordination:
Contrary to the belief that Lightsaber MMA is just theatrical, it offers intense physical training. The art form demands cardiovascular fitness, agility, and coordination. Practitioners develop a strong core, enhanced reflexes, and improved overall physical health, which are fundamental benefits of any martial art.

Mental Agility and Focus:
Lightsaber MMA is not just swinging a lightsaber; it involves strategic thinking and concentration. Practitioners learn to anticipate their opponent's moves, requiring mental agility and focus. This cognitive

training is practical in everyday life, enhancing one's ability to make quick decisions and remain focused under pressure.

Stress Relief and Emotional Balance:
Engaging in Lightsaber MMA provides an excellent outlet for stress. The physical exertion combined with the discipline required helps in releasing tension, promoting emotional balance. This aspect of mental health is often overlooked in the discussion of martial arts but is crucial in today's fast-paced world.

Self-Defense Skills:
While Lightsaber MMA may draw inspiration from a science fiction universe, the combat techniques are grounded in traditional martial arts. Practitioners learn valuable self-defense skills, including how to gauge distance and timing, and how to respond to an attack, making it a practical skill for personal safety.

Community and Social Interaction:
Lightsaber MMA brings together people from various backgrounds, creating a strong community bond. This social aspect is practical for mental health and well-being, as it fosters a sense of belonging and support.

Discipline and Personal Growth:
Like any martial art, Lightsaber MMA teaches discipline, perseverance, and respect. These life skills are invaluable and translate well beyond the training dojo into personal and professional life.

Adaptability and Inclusiveness:
Lightsaber MMA is adaptable to all ages and physical abilities, debunking the myth that it's exclusive or impractical for certain groups. Its inclusive nature makes it a practical choice for anyone interested in starting their martial arts journey.

Creative Expression and Confidence:
The practice encourages creative expression and individuality, which is essential for personal confidence and self-esteem. This aspect of Lightsaber MMA fosters personal growth and self-assurance, which are practical and beneficial in everyday life.

Lightsaber MMA is far from impractical. It offers a unique blend of physical fitness, mental sharpness, emotional well-being, and practical self-defense skills, all wrapped up in an engaging and dynamic package. It's a testament to the evolving nature of martial arts and its ability to adapt to modern interests while retaining its core benefits.

"Real-World Scenarios Where Lightsaber MMA Techniques Have Proven Effective"

In the evolving world of martial arts, Lightsaber MMA has made a significant impact, proving its effectiveness in various real-world scenarios. Here, I'll share some instances where the unique blend of traditional martial arts and lightsaber techniques has made a real difference.

Self-Defense:
Many practitioners have found Lightsaber MMA techniques to be highly effective in self-defense situations. The agility and reflexes developed through Lightsaber MMA training have helped individuals in real-life scenarios requiring quick thinking and rapid response. The art teaches not only physical defense maneuvers but also situational awareness, a crucial aspect of self-defense.

Physical Fitness and Rehabilitation:
In the realm of physical fitness and rehabilitation, Lightsaber MMA techniques offer a unique blend of cardio, strength training, and flexibility exercises. People recovering from injuries have used modified

Lightsaber MMA exercises as a form of physical therapy, aiding in their rehabilitation process while keeping the workouts engaging and enjoyable.

Stress Relief and Mental Health:
In today's fast-paced world, the mental health benefits of Lightsaber MMA cannot be overstated. Many individuals have found the practice to be an effective stress reliever, helping to manage anxiety and improve overall mental well-being. The focus required in Lightsaber MMA training fosters mindfulness, which is beneficial in alleviating stress.

Community Building and Social Interaction:
Lightsaber MMA has proven effective in building communities and enhancing social interaction. By training together, people from various backgrounds have formed strong bonds, fostering a sense of belonging and teamwork. This aspect of Lightsaber MMA goes beyond physical training, contributing to social well-being and community building.

Enhancing Concentration in Academics and Professional Life:
Students and professionals who practice Lightsaber MMA have reported improved concentration and focus in their academic and professional pursuits. The discipline and mental focus required in Lightsaber MMA training translate into better concentration and productivity in other areas of life.

Lightsaber MMA is more than just a form of martial arts; it's a comprehensive discipline that offers practical benefits in self-defense, physical fitness, mental health, community building, and personal development. Its real-world effectiveness is a testament to its growing popularity and the value it brings to practitioners' lives.

"Benefits of Training in a Martial Art that Combines Tradition with Modern Practicality, Such as Lightsaber MMA"

In the dynamic world of martial arts, the fusion of tradition with modern practicality, as seen in Lightsaber MMA, offers a multitude of transformative benefits, both personally and professionally. This blend creates a unique discipline that resonates with a broad audience, encompassing traditional martial arts enthusiasts and those seeking a contemporary, practical approach.

Holistic Development:
Lightsaber MMA offers a holistic approach to personal development. It combines the discipline, focus, and respect from traditional martial arts with the agility, creativity, and modern relevance of contemporary practices. This comprehensive development is crucial not just in martial arts but in all aspects of life.

Physical Health and Fitness:
Engaging in a martial art like Lightsaber MMA ensures a full-body workout. It enhances cardiovascular health, improves strength and flexibility, and promotes overall physical well-being. The dynamic nature of Lightsaber MMA, with its unique movements and sequences, makes fitness enjoyable and effective.

Mental Sharpness and Resilience:
Training in a martial art that requires quick thinking and adaptability, like Lightsaber MMA, sharpens the mind. It develops mental resilience, enhances focus, and fosters a growth mindset. These mental skills are invaluable in navigating life's challenges.

Stress Reduction and Emotional Wellness:
The practice of martial arts is a powerful stress reliever. The physical exertion coupled with focused training provides an effective outlet for stress and anxiety, leading to better emotional balance and overall

mental health.

Self-Defense Skills:
While Lightsaber MMA incorporates imaginative elements, the techniques and skills taught are grounded in practical self-defense. This training builds confidence in one's ability to protect themselves and others, which is a fundamental aspect of martial arts.

Enhanced Creativity and Problem Solving:
The creative and innovative aspects of Lightsaber MMA encourage out-of-the-box thinking. Practitioners learn to approach problems creatively, developing solutions that are effective both in and out of the dojo.

Cultural Appreciation and Diversity:
By blending traditional and modern elements, Lightsaber MMA fosters an appreciation for different cultures and practices. This exposure to diverse traditions and contemporary techniques enhances cultural understanding and acceptance.

Community and Social Engagement:
Lightsaber MMA attracts a diverse group of practitioners, creating a vibrant and inclusive community. Training in such an environment fosters social skills, builds friendships, and enhances one's sense of belonging.

Training in a martial art like Lightsaber MMA, which harmonizes traditional values with modern practicality, offers extensive benefits. It caters to the needs of those seeking a comprehensive, fulfilling, and practical approach to martial arts. This blend not only enhances physical and mental capabilities but also enriches emotional well-being and fosters a deep sense of community and cultural appreciation.

"Practicing Lightsaber MMA Techniques in Varied, Realistic Scenarios"

Embracing the world of Lightsaber Mixed Martial Arts (MMA) is more than just mastering the techniques; it's about applying these skills in varied, realistic scenarios. This practical application enhances the training experience, making it not only more engaging but also more effective in real-world situations.

Self-Defense Situations:

Practicing Lightsaber MMA techniques in self-defense scenarios is crucial. Through role-playing exercises, practitioners learn how to react in various situations, from warding off an attacker to protecting others. This training enhances situational awareness, decision-making under pressure, and the ability to use martial arts techniques effectively for defense.

Physical Fitness Challenges:

Incorporating Lightsaber MMA into fitness routines tests physical limits and endurance. For instance, obstacle courses that mimic real-life physical challenges can be integrated into training sessions. These exercises improve cardiovascular health, strength, agility, and stamina, making the practitioner more adept in handling physically demanding situations.

Mental and Emotional Resilience:

Realistic scenarios also include stress-inducing situations to train mental and emotional resilience. Techniques like controlled sparring in high-pressure environments help practitioners manage stress, maintain focus, and stay calm under pressure. This aspect of training is beneficial in daily life, enhancing one's ability to remain composed in challenging situations.

Teamwork and Leadership:

Group scenarios in Lightsaber MMA training foster teamwork and leadership skills. Practitioners learn to work together, strategize, and lead or follow as the situation demands. These skills are invaluable, translating into better team dynamics in professional and personal life.

Adaptation to Different Environments:

Training in varied environments – indoors, outdoors, in different weather conditions – prepares practitioners for any setting. This adaptability is a key aspect of martial arts, teaching practitioners to be versatile and resourceful.

Community and Social Interaction:

Engaging with the Lightsaber MMA community through public demonstrations or group training sessions enhances social interaction and public speaking skills. Practitioners learn to perform and communicate effectively in front of an audience, boosting confidence and social skills.

Practicing Lightsaber MMA techniques in varied, realistic scenarios is essential for a well-rounded training experience. It not only improves physical fitness and martial arts skills but also develops mental, emotional, and social abilities, preparing practitioners for real-world challenges. This holistic approach to training is what makes Lightsaber MMA an enriching and valuable martial art form.

CHAPTER FOUR

The Allure of Lightsaber MMA

Understanding the Appeal and Benefits
- The Captivating Blend of Tradition and Innovation
- Enhanced Physical and Mental Training
- The Modern Appeal: Engaging a New Generation
- Community Building and Social Interaction

Subsection: Understanding the Appeal and Benefits

1. *The Captivating Blend of Tradition and Innovation*

Step into the world of Lightsaber MMA, and you'll discover a captivating blend of time-honored martial arts traditions with the exhilarating innovation of lightsaber combat. This unique fusion not only preserves the core values of martial arts but also adds a layer of modern appeal that resonates with today's generation.

"Exploring How Lightsaber MMA Combines Traditional Martial Arts Principles with Innovative Techniques"

In the realm of martial arts, Lightsaber Mixed Martial Arts (MMA) emerges as a fascinating amalgamation of traditional martial arts principles and innovative techniques. This modern martial art form, inspired by the iconic imagery of lightsabers from the Star Wars universe, offers a unique training experience that is both rooted in the rich heritage of traditional martial arts and forward-thinking in its approach.

Fusion of Styles:
Lightsaber MMA is not confined to the boundaries of a single martial arts style. It is a fusion of various disciplines, ranging from Kenjutsu and Western Fencing to Dao, Wushu, and even Capoeira. This blend of styles creates a versatile and comprehensive martial arts system that offers depth and variety in training.

Emphasis on Traditional Values:
Despite its modern and imaginative flair, Lightsaber MMA upholds the traditional martial arts values of discipline, respect, and self-improvement. These core principles are integral to the training, ensuring that practitioners not only develop their physical skills but also grow in character and virtue.

Innovative Techniques and Adaptability:
Lightsaber MMA is characterized by its adaptability and the incorporation of innovative techniques. From acrobatic movements inspired by Wushu and Capoeira to the strategic approaches of Kenjutsu and fencing, Lightsaber MMA offers a dynamic and ever-evolving training experience.

Physical and Mental Conditioning:

The training in Lightsaber MMA is both physically demanding and mentally stimulating. Practitioners engage in exercises that improve strength, agility, and endurance, while also developing strategic thinking and mental resilience. This holistic approach to training ensures a balanced development of both body and mind.

Self-Defense Applications:

While Lightsaber MMA is inspired by a fictional weapon, the techniques taught have practical self-defense applications. The training emphasizes reflex development, spatial awareness, and effective response strategies that are applicable in real-world self-defense scenarios.

Community and Culture:

Lightsaber MMA fosters a strong sense of community among its practitioners. This martial arts form attracts a diverse group of enthusiasts, creating a melting pot of cultures and backgrounds. The community aspect of Lightsaber MMA contributes significantly to the learning experience, as practitioners share knowledge, techniques, and experiences.

Lightsaber MMA stands as a testament to the evolving nature of martial arts. It successfully bridges the gap between tradition and innovation, offering a martial arts experience that is both deeply rooted in classical principles and boldly imaginative in its approach. Through its diverse range of styles, emphasis on traditional values, innovative techniques, and community culture, Lightsaber MMA provides a unique and enriching path for personal growth and martial arts proficiency.

"Stories of Practitioners Who Found Renewed Passion for Martial Arts Through Lightsaber MMA"

In the world of martial arts, Lightsaber Mixed Martial Arts (MMA) has ignited a new wave of enthusiasm and passion. It's a modern take that combines the traditional aspects of martial arts with the exciting world of lightsaber combat. Let's explore some inspiring stories of individuals who rediscovered their love for martial arts through Lightsaber MMA.

Vicky's Journey from Burnout to Renewal:
Vicky, a long-time karate practitioner, faced a point where her martial arts journey had become stagnant. The routines felt monotonous, and her passion was fading. This changed when she discovered Lightsaber MMA. The innovative blend of traditional martial arts techniques with the dynamic and imaginative lightsaber combat rekindled her passion. She found new challenges and excitement in the art form, which not only revived her interest in martial arts but also added a new dimension to her skills.

Todd's Escape from the Mundane:
Todd, a software engineer, had never practiced martial arts. His life was mostly work, and he longed for an escape from the mundane. When he joined a Lightsaber MMA class, he found more than just a hobby; he discovered a community and a newfound passion. The classes offered him a perfect blend of physical exercise, mental discipline, and a touch of childhood nostalgia. Lightsaber MMA became his gateway into the broader world of martial arts, leading him to explore other forms as well.

Emma's Confidence Boost:
Emma, a teenager struggling with self-esteem issues, was initially skeptical about martial arts. Her perception changed when she saw a Lightsaber MMA demonstration at her school. Intrigued by the grace

and strength of the practitioners, she decided to give it a try. The inclusive environment and the empowering nature of the art form gave her confidence a significant boost. She became more outgoing and self-assured, both in and out of the dojo.

John's Return to Martial Arts:

John, a retired military veteran, had a background in mixed martial arts but had drifted away from practice over the years. Discovering Lightsaber MMA gave him a reason to return. The art form's blend of discipline, physicality, and the fun element associated with lightsabers appealed to him. It provided a familiar grounding in martial arts while offering something new and exciting to master.

Linda's Path to Healing:

After a personal tragedy, Linda found herself at a loss, struggling to find something that brought joy. Her son, a fan of Star Wars, suggested they try Lightsaber MMA together. This experience was transformative for Linda. It became a therapeutic outlet, helping her to cope with her grief. The physical activity, combined with the supportive community, played a crucial role in her healing process.

These stories highlight the unique impact of Lightsaber MMA in reigniting passion for martial arts. It's a testament to how this innovative art form is appealing to a broad spectrum of people, offering a fresh perspective on traditional martial arts and providing a platform for personal growth, healing, and community building. Whether you're a seasoned martial artist or a newcomer, Lightsaber MMA has something to offer – a chance to connect with your passion, challenge yourself, and be part of an inspiring community.

"The Power of Blending Traditional and Modern Martial Arts: Increased Engagement and Skill Diversity"

In the world of personal development and martial arts, there's an incredible power in blending traditional disciplines with modern innovations. This fusion, epitomized by practices like Lightsaber MMA, brings forth a plethora of benefits, including increased engagement and a rich diversity of skills. Let's delve into how this blend transforms the martial arts experience.

Revitalizing Traditional Martial Arts:

Integrating modern elements into traditional martial arts breathes new life into these age-old practices. For many, traditional martial arts can feel distant or rigid. By infusing contemporary techniques and philosophies, like those found in Lightsaber MMA, these practices become more relatable and engaging for today's practitioners. This revitalization attracts a broader audience, from young enthusiasts to those seeking a modern twist on martial arts training.

Enhanced Physical and Mental Engagement:

The blend of traditional and modern martial arts requires both physical and mental agility. Traditional martial arts focus on discipline, technique, and precision, while modern styles often emphasize speed, adaptability, and creativity. This combination ensures that practitioners are not just physically engaged but also mentally stimulated, making each training session a comprehensive workout for the body and mind.

Diversity of Skills and Techniques:

The fusion of different martial arts styles results in a rich tapestry of skills and techniques. Practitioners are exposed to a wide range of movements, from the calculated strikes of Karate to the fluidity of Brazilian Jiu-Jitsu and the theatrical flair of Lightsaber MMA. This diversity not only enhances one's martial arts repertoire but also fosters a deeper understanding and appreciation of different martial arts cultures and philosophies.

Increased Accessibility and Inclusivity:

By blending various martial arts styles, these practices become more accessible and inclusive. Traditional martial arts can sometimes be intimidating or seem unapproachable. The incorporation of modern elements, familiar to a wider audience, breaks down barriers and creates a welcoming environment for people of all ages, backgrounds, and skill levels.

Building a Holistic Martial Artist:

The comprehensive nature of this blend ensures the development of a holistic martial artist. Practitioners benefit from the discipline and respect ingrained in traditional martial arts, while also embracing the flexibility, creativity, and practical self-defense skills offered by modern techniques. This well-rounded approach prepares individuals not just for martial arts competitions but for real-life challenges as well.

Fostering a Community of Diverse Practitioners:

The diversity in training attracts a wide range of individuals, creating a melting pot of practitioners. This community aspect is vital, as it allows for the sharing of knowledge, experiences, and cultural perspectives. In such an environment, learning is not just about techniques; it's also about understanding and respecting different viewpoints and backgrounds.

The blend of traditional and modern martial arts, exemplified by practices like Lightsaber MMA, offers numerous benefits. It revitalizes martial arts training, increases physical and mental engagement, diversifies skills, enhances accessibility, and builds a community of diverse practitioners. This fusion approach not only makes martial arts more relevant and exciting but also molds practitioners into well-rounded individuals equipped with a diverse set of skills to navigate life's challenges.

Seek out lightsaber MMA classes or demonstrations to experience this blend firsthand.

2. Enhanced Physical and Mental Training

Lightsaber MMA is not just a visually stunning art; it's a comprehensive training system that enhances both physical and mental faculties. It goes beyond the conventional to offer a well-rounded approach to fitness and cognitive development.

"Mastering the Art of Lightsaber Combat: The Rigors of Physical Training"

Embarking on the journey of mastering Lightsaber combat in the realm of Mixed Martial Arts is a testament to the rigorous physical training and discipline required. This modern martial art form, inspired by the iconic imagery of lightsabers from the Star Wars saga, offers an exhilarating and demanding path to physical mastery and personal growth.

Intensive Cardiovascular Training:
The foundation of Lightsaber combat is intensive cardiovascular training. Practitioners engage in various high-intensity workouts that increase heart rate and build stamina. This endurance is crucial, as Lightsaber combat involves rapid movements, quick reflexes, and prolonged physical exertion. Cardiovascular fitness not only enhances performance

in the dojo but also contributes to overall heart health and stamina.

Strength and Conditioning:

Lightsaber combat demands a significant level of strength. Training involves a regimen of weightlifting, bodyweight exercises, and resistance training to build muscle strength, particularly in the arms, shoulders, and core. This strength is vital for wielding the lightsaber effectively, allowing for powerful strikes and solid defense. Conditioning the body in this way prepares practitioners for the physical demands of Lightsaber combat and reduces the risk of injury.

Agility and Flexibility Training:

Agility and flexibility are cornerstones of Lightsaber combat. The art form requires quick, agile movements and the ability to maneuver with grace and precision. Practitioners often engage in activities like yoga, pilates, and dynamic stretching to enhance flexibility. This training improves range of motion, balance, and coordination, all of which are essential in mastering the art of Lightsaber combat.

Reflex and Reaction Time Development:

A key aspect of Lightsaber combat is developing quick reflexes and reaction time. Training includes exercises that enhance sensory awareness and response time, such as sparring, reaction drills, and reflex conditioning. The ability to anticipate and react swiftly is crucial in Lightsaber combat, mirroring the quick decision-making required in real-life situations.

Mental Fortitude and Focus:

While physically demanding, Lightsaber combat also requires mental fortitude and focus. Practitioners learn to maintain concentration amidst physical exertion, a skill that translates into improved mental resilience in everyday life. The mental aspect of training involves meditation, visualization techniques, and mindfulness practices.

Technical Skill Development:
Mastering Lightsaber combat involves learning and refining technical skills. This includes understanding the mechanics of Lightsaber handling, mastering various combat forms, and perfecting striking and blocking techniques. Continuous practice and refinement of these skills are necessary for proficiency in Lightsaber combat.

Endurance and Perseverance:
Perhaps the most critical aspect of training in Lightsaber combat is developing endurance and perseverance. The path to mastery is challenging and requires sustained effort, dedication, and resilience. This journey instills a sense of perseverance that practitioners carry with them in all aspects of life.

Mastering Lightsaber combat in Mixed Martial Arts is a rigorous and transformative journey that extends beyond physical training. It embodies a holistic approach to personal development, encompassing cardiovascular fitness, strength, agility, mental fortitude, technical skill, and enduring perseverance. This journey not only prepares practitioners for the physical demands of Lightsaber combat but also equips them with life skills that transcend the dojo. As they embark on this path, they embrace a journey of continual growth, challenge, and self-discovery.

"Harnessing Mental Agility and Strategic Thinking through Lightsaber MMA"

In the expansive universe of martial arts, Lightsaber Mixed Martial Arts (MMA) stands out not only for its physical rigor but also for its profound impact on mental agility and strategic thinking. As a transformative practice, it extends beyond the physical realm, engaging the mind in ways that are both challenging and exhilarating. Let's explore how Lightsaber MMA catalyzes sharpening mental faculties and enhancing strategic acumen.

Cultivating Focus and Concentration:
The art of Lightsaber MMA requires an unparalleled level of focus and concentration. Practitioners learn to channel their thoughts, filter distractions, and direct their attention to the task at hand. This intense focus is crucial during combat, where a momentary lapse can mean the difference between a successful strike and a missed opportunity. The ability to concentrate under pressure translates into improved focus in everyday life, enhancing productivity and efficiency.

Strategic Planning and Execution:
Engaging in Lightsaber MMA combat is akin to playing a high-speed, physical game of chess. Each movement and decision must be strategic, anticipating the opponent's next move while planning your own. Practitioners develop the skill to think several steps ahead, considering multiple potential outcomes and choosing the most effective course of action. This strategic planning and execution are invaluable skills, applicable in personal and professional scenarios where strategic decision-making is key.

Enhancing Quick Thinking and Adaptability:
In the dynamic environment of Lightsaber MMA, situations can change rapidly. Practitioners learn to think on their feet, making swift decisions in response to their opponent's actions. This ability to quickly analyze and adapt is a testament to the mental agility developed through Lightsaber MMA. It fosters a mindset that is flexible, resilient, and capable of navigating through life's unexpected turns.

Building Emotional Intelligence:
Martial arts, at their core, are about self-mastery, and Lightsaber MMA is no exception. Practitioners engage in exercises that challenge not only their physical abilities but also their emotional responses. They learn to manage emotions like frustration, anger, and fear, transforming these feelings into focused determination. This emotional intelligence

is crucial for maintaining mental clarity and making reasoned decisions under stress.

Promoting Mind-Body Coordination:

Lightsaber MMA necessitates a high degree of mind-body coordination. Practitioners must be acutely aware of their physical movements while maintaining a strategic mindset. This synchronization of mind and body enhances overall coordination, a skill that extends beyond martial arts to improve general motor skills and physical responsiveness.

Fostering Creative Problem Solving:

The imaginative aspect of Lightsaber MMA encourages creative thinking. Practitioners are often faced with scenarios that require innovative solutions, pushing them to think outside the box. This creativity in problem-solving is a crucial aspect of strategic thinking, enabling individuals to approach challenges from unique perspectives and find novel solutions.

Encouraging Continuous Learning and Growth:

Finally, Lightsaber MMA instills a mindset of continuous learning and growth. The art form is ever-evolving, and practitioners must stay open to new techniques and strategies. This mindset of lifelong learning and adaptability is crucial for mental agility, as it keeps the mind active, curious, and always ready to absorb new information.

Lightsaber MMA offers a unique platform for developing mental agility and strategic thinking. Its blend of physical engagement and mental challenge creates a comprehensive training environment that sharpens the mind, enhances strategic acumen, and prepares practitioners for the complex challenges of life. This martial art form is not just about wielding a lightsaber; it's about mastering the art of strategic thinking and mental resilience.

"Unleashing Potential: The Fitness and Cognitive Benefits of Integrated Martial Arts Training"

In the journey towards personal growth and mastery, the integration of various martial arts forms, including the innovative Lightsaber MMA, offers a unique pathway. This amalgamation not only revolutionizes physical fitness but also enhances cognitive abilities, unlocking new dimensions of personal development. Let's dive deep into the myriad benefits of this integrated training.

Holistic Physical Fitness:

Integrated martial arts training, such as Lightsaber MMA, offers a full-body workout that transcends the typical gym routine. This form of training combines cardiovascular endurance, strength building, flexibility, and agility work. Practitioners experience improved muscle tone, enhanced stamina, and better overall physical conditioning. Unlike traditional workouts, this dynamic approach keeps the body constantly challenged, leading to more significant and sustained fitness results.

Enhanced Cognitive Functioning:

The mental benefits of martial arts are profound. Training in disciplines like Lightsaber MMA requires constant mental engagement – from remembering complex sequences to strategizing in real-time during sparring sessions. This mental gymnastics enhances memory, sharpens focus, and boosts problem-solving skills. Regular practice leads to improved neural pathways, making practitioners more alert and mentally agile in their everyday lives.

Stress Relief and Emotional Regulation:

Engaging in martial arts is an effective stress reliever. The physical exertion releases endorphins, the body's natural mood elevators, leading to a sense of well-being and tranquility. Moreover, the discipline required in martial arts fosters emotional regulation. Practitioners learn to channel their emotions constructively, a skill that is invaluable in managing the stresses of daily life.

Increased Mind-Body Coordination:

Integrated martial arts training necessitates a high degree of mind-body coordination. Practices like Lightsaber MMA require practitioners to be acutely aware of their movements while maintaining strategic thinking. This synchronization enhances overall coordination, improves reaction times, and cultivates a heightened sense of spatial awareness, benefiting both physical and cognitive aspects of daily activities.

Boost in Confidence and Self-Efficacy:

The journey through martial arts is filled with milestones and achievements. Each new skill mastered and each challenge overcome contributes to a growing sense of confidence and self-efficacy. This boost in self-esteem extends beyond the dojo, empowering individuals in their personal and professional lives.

Promotion of Lifelong Learning and Adaptability:

The ever-evolving nature of integrated martial arts, especially with modern forms like Lightsaber MMA, encourages a mindset of lifelong learning. Practitioners are constantly adapting to new techniques and scenarios, fostering a mindset that is flexible, open to change, and always ready for growth.

Social Interaction and Community Building:

Integrated martial arts training is often a communal activity. Practitioners learn from each other, share experiences, and support one another's growth. This sense of community is not only motivational but also instrumental in building social skills and fostering connections.

The fusion of traditional and modern martial arts training offers a comprehensive platform for physical and cognitive development. The holistic approach of disciplines like Lightsaber MMA not only cultivates a fit body and a sharp mind but also nurtures emotional well-being, self-confidence, and a sense of community. This integrated training is a powerful tool in the quest for personal excellence, encapsulating the essence of self-improvement and empowerment.

"Elevating Your Workout Regime: The Transformative Power of Lightsaber Drills and Sparring"

Imagine transforming your regular workout routine into an invigorating, holistic experience that not only challenges your body but also stimulates your mind and spirit. This is the power of incorporating Lightsaber drills and sparring into your fitness regime. As an advocate for innovative and effective methods of self-improvement, I believe that integrating these dynamic elements can unlock new levels of personal growth and physical prowess.

Enhanced Cardiovascular Fitness:
Integrating Lightsaber drills into your workout significantly boosts cardiovascular health. These high-energy routines require sustained movement, which elevates the heart rate and improves blood circulation. Regular Lightsaber training sessions are a fun and engaging way to enhance heart health, increase lung capacity, and reduce the risk of heart-related conditions.

Improved Strength and Endurance:
Lightsaber sparring is a full-body workout that builds muscular strength and endurance. The combat sequences engage different muscle groups, from the core to the arms and legs, providing a balanced strength-training exercise. This form of functional fitness not only tones your muscles but also enhances endurance, ensuring you're fit and ready to tackle everyday physical challenges.

Agility and Reflex Development:

The quick movements and rapid reflexes required in Lightsaber sparring foster agility. Practitioners learn to maneuver swiftly, enhancing their reaction time and coordination. This agility training is beneficial not just in martial arts but in various sports and daily activities, where quick reflexes and coordinated movements are essential.

Mental Focus and Concentration:

Lightsaber training requires a high degree of mental focus and concentration. The need to anticipate an opponent's moves and respond strategically enhances cognitive abilities. This mental discipline translates into improved concentration and focus in other areas of life, boosting productivity and problem-solving skills.

Stress Relief and Emotional Balance:

Engaging in Lightsaber drills is an excellent stress reliever. The physical exertion releases endorphins, the body's natural mood elevators, promoting relaxation and emotional well-being. The meditative aspect of mastering the movements also helps in achieving mental clarity and emotional balance.

Enhanced Self-Defense Skills:

While Lightsaber MMA is inspired by the fictional universe of Star Wars, the combat techniques have practical self-defense applications. Practitioners learn valuable defensive maneuvers, enhancing their ability to protect themselves in real-life situations.

Building Self-Confidence and Empowerment:

There's a unique sense of accomplishment and empowerment that comes with mastering Lightsaber drills and sparring techniques. This process builds self-confidence, as practitioners witness their progress and capabilities. The confidence gained in the dojo permeates other aspects of life, empowering individuals to tackle challenges with a positive mindset.

Community and Social Interaction:
Lightsaber training often occurs in a group setting, fostering a sense of community and belonging. Practitioners share a common interest and passion, leading to meaningful connections and friendships. This social interaction is integral to mental health, providing a supportive network that enriches the training experience.

Incorporating Lightsaber drills and sparring into your regular workouts offers a myriad of benefits, transcending traditional exercise regimes. It's an innovative approach to fitness that combines physical prowess with mental sharpness, emotional well-being, and a sense of community. Embrace this dynamic form of training, and experience a transformation in your workout routine that goes beyond physical boundaries, leading to holistic growth and empowerment.

3. The Modern Appeal: Engaging a New Generation

The allure of Lightsaber MMA lies in its ability to engage a new generation of martial artists. Its modern twist, rooted in popular culture, attracts individuals who might not have been drawn to traditional martial arts.

"Igniting the Passion in the Tech-Savvy Generation: The Allure of Lightsaber MMA"

In today's fast-paced, technology-driven world, engaging the younger, tech-savvy, and visually oriented generation can be a challenge. However, Lightsaber Mixed Martial Arts (MMA) has emerged as a captivating and effective way to connect with this demographic. This modern martial art, inspired by the futuristic elegance of lightsabers, is more than just a physical discipline; it's a bridge between traditional martial arts and the digital age. Let's explore why Lightsaber MMA has become particularly appealing to this younger generation.

Visual and Technological Appeal:
Lightsaber MMA resonates with the younger generation's penchant for visual stimulation and technological advancements. The vibrant glow of the lightsabers, combined with the dynamic movements, creates a visually engaging experience that captures the imagination. This generation, raised with video games and CGI movies, finds a connection with the visually appealing and technologically advanced nature of Lightsaber MMA.

Fusion of Fantasy and Reality:
The world of Lightsaber MMA blurs the lines between fantasy and reality, something that deeply resonates with a generation fascinated by virtual worlds and sci-fi themes. It offers an opportunity to live out the adventures they've seen in movies and video games, blending their digital experiences with physical activity uniquely and excitingly.

Social Media and Community Building:
The rise of social media has created a platform for sharing experiences and building communities. Lightsaber MMA, with its visual appeal and unique nature, is highly shareable content. Young practitioners are drawn to this community aspect, where they can showcase their skills, connect with like-minded individuals, and be part of a global community.

Interactive and Engaging Training:
The training involved in Lightsaber MMA is interactive and engaging, keeping pace with the fast-moving, high-stimulation environment the younger generation is accustomed to. The classes often integrate

music, lights, and other elements that make the training session more than just a workout – it's an experience.

Empowerment and Confidence Building:
Lightsaber MMA offers a path to empowerment and confidence-building. The younger generation, navigating the complexities of growing up in a digital world, finds a sense of achievement and self-assuredness in mastering the art. The discipline, focus, and physical skills developed through Lightsaber MMA training translate into increased confidence in other areas of their lives.

Physical Fitness in a Digital Era:
With the increasing concern about sedentary lifestyles prevalent among the younger generation, Lightsaber MMA offers an innovative solution. It combines physical fitness with an element of fun and engagement, encouraging more young people to step away from their screens and engage in physical activity.

Mental Health and Stress Relief:
In a world where young people are facing unprecedented levels of stress and mental health challenges, Lightsaber MMA provides a much-needed outlet. The physical exertion, combined with the discipline and focus required, serves as a stress reliever and contributes to better mental health.

Lightsaber MMA presents a unique and effective way to engage the tech-savvy, visually-oriented younger generation. It offers a perfect blend of physical fitness, mental discipline, and technological appeal, wrapped in a visually stimulating package. By tapping into their love for technology and visual media, Lightsaber MMA not only promotes physical well-being but also provides a platform for personal growth, community building, and empowerment.

"Igniting a New Generation: How Lightsaber MMA Sparked a Martial Arts Revolution"

In my journey as an instructor of Lightsaber MMA, I've encountered countless stories of transformation and discovery. Among these, the tales of young practitioners who found their passion for martial arts through Lightsaber MMA stand out. These stories are not just about physical training; they're about finding a calling, a source of inspiration, and a path to personal growth.

Landon's Journey of Self-Discovery:
Landon, a 16-year-old high school student, had always felt disconnected from traditional sports. Everything changed when he saw a Lightsaber MMA demonstration at a local event. The energy, the movement, the blend of artistry and athleticism immediately captivated him. Landon found Lightsaber MMA a platform that combined his love for technology and movement. It became more than a hobby; it was a way for him to express himself, to belong, to grow. Through his training, Landon developed not just physical strength but also a newfound confidence that spilled over into every aspect of his life.

Brianna's Tale of Empowerment:
Brianna, a young woman in her early twenties, struggled with self-esteem issues. She stumbled upon a Lightsaber MMA class almost by accident. The first time she held the lightsaber, she felt a sense of power and control she had never experienced before. Each session helped her not only to improve her physical fitness but also to build her mental strength. In Lightsaber MMA, she found a supportive community that celebrated her progress, respected her journey, and empowered her to push her limits. This newfound strength transformed Brianna, giving her the courage to face challenges beyond the dojo.

Lucas's Path to Focus and Discipline:
Lucas, a teenager known for his restless energy and lack of focus, was introduced to Lightsaber MMA by his parents in hopes of channeling his energy positively. Initially skeptical, Lucas quickly became enamored with the discipline, structure, and creativity of the art form. Lightsaber MMA provided an outlet for his boundless energy and a framework for channeling it constructively. As he advanced in his training, his focus and discipline improved, which was reflected in his academic performance and personal relationships.

Mikah's Breakthrough from Digital to Physical:
In a world where digital interactions often outweigh physical activities, Mikah's story stands as a testament to the power of engaging in a tangible, physical practice. A confessed 'gamer', Mikah found a real-world connection to her digital interests through Lightsaber MMA. The art form's resemblance to the virtual worlds she loved provided an initial draw, but she soon discovered deeper benefits. The physical engagement, the rhythm of the fights, and the tactical thinking involved in sparring mirrored the strategic challenges she enjoyed in video games, but with added physical and social benefits.

These stories from young practitioners underscore the unique appeal of Lightsaber MMA. It resonates with the tech-savvy, visually-oriented younger generation by combining elements of fantasy and reality, offering a physically and mentally engaging experience. Lightsaber MMA serves as a bridge, drawing them into the world of martial arts and providing a platform for physical fitness, personal growth, and community building. By tapping into their passions and interests, Lightsaber MMA lights a spark that can ignite a lifelong journey in martial arts and self-discovery.

"Revitalizing Martial Arts in the Digital Age: The Impact of Lightsaber MMA"

In this digital era, where virtual experiences often eclipse the allure of physical activities, the relevance and appeal of traditional martial arts face a new challenge. However, the emergence of Lightsaber Mixed Martial Arts (MMA) has played a pivotal role in reinvigorating interest in martial arts, making it resonate with the digital generation. This innovative discipline blends the timeless principles of martial arts with the captivating allure of a modern, visually dynamic practice.

Bridging Traditional and Modern Worlds:
Lightsaber MMA serves as a bridge between the traditional world of martial arts and the digital age. It retains the core values and disciplines of traditional martial arts, such as respect, discipline, and physical mastery, while infusing them with a contemporary twist that appeals to the tech-savvy generation. This blend creates a unique platform that is both rooted in history and relevant to today's digital landscape.

Visual Appeal and Engagement:
The visual aspect of Lightsaber MMA is undeniably captivating. The use of lightsabers, with their vibrant colors and futuristic appeal, resonates deeply with a generation raised on digital imagery and sci-fi movies. This visual engagement is crucial in attracting young enthusiasts who might otherwise be more inclined towards virtual experiences than physical training.

Incorporating Digital Elements in Training:
The incorporation of digital technology in Lightsaber MMA training adds another layer of appeal. Many training centers use apps, virtual reality, and other digital tools to enhance the learning experience. This integration of technology in training not only makes the practice more appealing but also more accessible, allowing practitioners to engage

with martial arts in a medium they are comfortable and familiar with.

Fostering Community in a Digital World:
Lightsaber MMA has harnessed the power of digital platforms to build a global community. Social media groups, online forums, and virtual events allow practitioners from around the world to connect, share experiences, and learn from each other. This sense of community is vital in keeping martial arts relevant, providing a space where enthusiasts can gather, regardless of their geographical location.

Adapting to Modern Fitness Trends:
The physical training involved in Lightsaber MMA aligns with modern fitness trends, emphasizing holistic well-being, agility, and mental fitness. This alignment makes it an attractive option for those seeking a workout that is both physically challenging and mentally stimulating, combining the best of fitness and martial arts training.

Promoting Mindful Use of Technology:
Lightsaber MMA encourages a mindful approach to technology. While it leverages digital tools and appeals to a tech-savvy audience, it also emphasizes the importance of physical activity, interpersonal connections, and being present in the moment. This balance is crucial in an age where the digital world can often be overwhelming.

Inspiring the Next Generation:
Perhaps most importantly, Lightsaber MMA plays a significant role in inspiring the next generation of martial artists. By offering an exciting, accessible, and relevant entry point into the world of martial arts, it paves the way for young individuals to explore deeper aspects of martial arts culture and history.

Lightsaber MMA represents a dynamic evolution in the world of martial arts, perfectly poised to maintain its relevance and appeal in the digital age. It stands as a testament to the enduring power of martial arts, adapting and evolving to meet the needs and interests of a new generation while preserving its rich heritage and values. This innovative discipline not only keeps martial arts relevant but also ensures its continued growth and popularity in our rapidly changing world.

"Igniting Young Minds: The Transformative Power of Lightsaber MMA in Schools and Youth Programs"

I've always emphasized the importance of engaging and empowering our youth. Introducing Lightsaber Mixed Martial Arts (MMA) into schools and youth programs is a groundbreaking way to connect with the younger generation, igniting their passion for physical activity and personal growth. Let's delve into the goals and benefits of this innovative approach.

Cultivating Physical Fitness in a Digital Era:

In a time where screen time often supersedes physical activity, Lightsaber MMA offers an exciting alternative. The goal is to draw students away from passive digital consumption and encourage active, physical engagement. This practice promotes cardiovascular health, improves strength and flexibility, and instills a habit of regular exercise – a crucial counterbalance to the sedentary lifestyle prevalent among today's youth.

Fostering Discipline and Focus:

One of the core benefits of martial arts, including Lightsaber MMA, is the development of discipline and focus. These skills are essential in academic and personal life. The structured nature of martial arts training teaches students the value of commitment, practice, and perseverance, helping them to apply these principles to their studies and other life pursuits.

Enhancing Mental Well-being:

Physical activity, particularly martial arts, is known to improve mental well-being. Lightsaber MMA, with its dynamic and immersive nature, serves as a stress reliever and confidence booster. It also offers a constructive outlet for youthful energy and emotions, aiding in emotional regulation and resilience – vital skills in navigating the complexities of adolescence.

Building Social Skills and Community:

Incorporating Lightsaber MMA into youth programs creates a sense of community and belonging. It encourages teamwork, communication, and mutual respect among peers. These social interactions foster a sense of inclusion and help students develop essential interpersonal skills, preparing them for collaborative environments in the future.

Encouraging Creativity and Self-expression:

Lightsaber MMA is not just a physical discipline; it's an art form that allows for creativity and self-expression. The combination of traditional martial arts with the imaginative aspect of lightsaber combat provides a unique avenue for students to express themselves, encouraging creative thinking and innovation.

Developing Tactical Thinking and Problem-solving:

Martial arts training, especially in a format like Lightsaber MMA, involves strategic thinking and quick decision-making. These practices enhance cognitive abilities such as problem-solving, tactical thinking, and spatial awareness. Such skills are transferable to academic settings, enhancing students' learning and comprehension abilities.

Instilling a Lifelong Love for Learning and Growth:

The ultimate goal of introducing Lightsaber MMA in schools and youth programs is to instill a lifelong love for learning and personal growth. It teaches students that progress comes with practice and patience, fostering a growth mindset that views challenges as opportunities for development.

Bridging Generational Gaps through Shared Interests:
Lightsaber MMA bridges the gap between generations. It connects with the youth through a medium they find fascinating while rooted in the timeless principles of martial arts. This shared interest fosters understanding and connection between instructors and students, and even between parents and children.

Introducing Lightsaber MMA in schools and youth programs is a powerful tool for engaging the younger audience. It offers a multifaceted approach to development, encompassing physical fitness, mental well-being, social skills, and cognitive growth. We can ignite a passion for lifelong learning and self-improvement in our youth, setting them on a path to becoming well-rounded, empowered individuals.

4. Community Building and Social Interaction

Beyond individual training, lightsaber MMA fosters a strong sense of community and provides ample opportunities for social interaction. This aspect is integral to its growing popularity and appeal.

"Uniting Through Lightsaber MMA: Building Vibrant, Supportive Communities"

In my years of coaching and speaking, I've witnessed the incredible power of community. Lightsaber Mixed Martial Arts (MMA) classes and events epitomize this power, creating vibrant, supportive communities that go beyond physical fitness. Let's explore the profound impact these gatherings have on individuals and groups alike, fostering connections, growth, and shared experiences.

A Shared Passion as a Unifying Force:

Lightsaber MMA brings together individuals from diverse backgrounds, united by their passion for martial arts and the iconic symbol of the lightsaber. This shared interest forms the foundation of a community where members feel a strong sense of belonging and identity. It's a space where enthusiasts, irrespective of age or background, connect over a common love, breaking down barriers and fostering inclusivity.

Empathy and Support in Learning:

The learning environment in Lightsaber MMA classes is imbued with empathy and support. Beginners and advanced practitioners alike are welcomed with encouragement. As participants face challenges and celebrate successes together, a bond of mutual respect and support forms. This environment nurtures not only skill development but also personal growth, as individuals learn to empathize with and uplift each other.

Cultivating Leadership and Mentorship:

Lightsaber MMA communities naturally foster leadership and mentorship. More experienced practitioners often take on mentorship roles, guiding newcomers. This leadership development is integral to community building, as it encourages a culture of passing on knowledge, skills, and values. Through mentorship, members find purpose and fulfillment, enhancing the community's strength and resilience.

Enhancing Social Interaction and Networking:

Classes and events offer opportunities for social interaction, extending beyond the realm of martial arts. They become networking hubs where people share experiences, advice, and form friendships. This social aspect is particularly valuable in our increasingly digital world, offering a space for genuine, face-to-face connections.

A Platform for Celebrating Diversity:

Lightsaber MMA events are a melting pot of cultures and perspectives, celebrating diversity. They provide a platform for individuals to express their unique backgrounds and stories, enriching the community with a tapestry of experiences. This celebration of diversity not only enhances cultural understanding but also adds depth and color to the community.

Fostering a Sense of Achievement and Pride:

Participating in Lightsaber MMA events, whether as a competitor or a supporter, instills a sense of achievement and pride. Collective participation in tournaments or demonstrations strengthens community bonds as members cheer for each other, share in victories, and offer comfort in defeats. These shared experiences build a strong, interconnected community.

Community Service and Outreach:

Many Lightsaber MMA communities engage in outreach and service, extending their impact beyond their immediate circle. Whether it's organizing charity events or offering free classes to underprivileged groups, these acts of service reinforce the community's values and its commitment to making a positive difference in the world.

Digital Platforms for Continuous Connection:

Utilizing digital platforms, Lightsaber MMA communities stay connected beyond physical meetings. Social media groups, online forums, and virtual events ensure that the sense of community is sustained. These digital connections are particularly significant in times when physical gatherings might not be possible, providing a space for continuous engagement, learning, and support.

Lightsaber MMA classes and events are more than just avenues for physical training; they are catalysts for creating vibrant, supportive communities. These communities play a crucial role in personal development, offering a sense of belonging, mutual support, and shared joy. They exemplify the power of unity and collective growth, reminding us that together, we can achieve more than we ever could alone. As we foster and participate in such communities, we contribute to a world that is more connected, empathetic, and empowered.

"The Bonds Forged in Lightsaber MMA: A Tale of Friendship and Connection"

I've witnessed countless stories of transformation, growth, and connection. Among these, the friendships and connections formed through Lightsaber Mixed Martial Arts (MMA) stand out as powerful testaments to the unifying power of shared passions and challenges. Let me share with you some personal anecdotes that highlight the profound impact of Lightsaber MMA on building lasting relationships.

The Story of Billy and Sue:
At a Lightsaber MMA workshop, I met Billy and Sue, two individuals from vastly different backgrounds. Billy, a quiet graphic designer, and Sue, an exuberant college student, found common ground in their love for martial arts and science fiction. Through their training, they formed a bond that transcended the dojo. They supported each other through each bout, celebrating victories and learning from defeats. Their friendship developed into a deep mutual respect and understanding, illustrating how Lightsaber MMA can bring people together, fostering connections that last a lifetime.

The Journey of The Weekend Warriors:
I remember a group fondly referred to as "The Weekend Warriors," a diverse mix of individuals who met every Saturday for Lightsaber

MMA practice. They were accountants, teachers, students, and more, united by their enthusiasm for Lightsaber combat. The dojo became a melting pot where age, profession, and background faded into the background, replaced by camaraderie and shared goals. They not only sparred together but also shared life stories and advice, turning their weekend sessions into a much-anticipated gathering of friends.

The Bond Between Instructor and Student:

As a Lightsaber MMA instructor, I've formed unique bonds with my students. One such connection was with a young man named Justin. Initially, he was reserved and hesitant, but as he grew in skill and confidence, our relationship evolved. We shared not just techniques and drills, but also life lessons and personal growth stories. This bond between instructor and student is a testament to the mentorship and guidance inherent in martial arts training, going beyond physical prowess to encompass personal development.

The Family That Trains Together:

One of the most heartwarming stories comes from a family that joined Lightsaber MMA together. The Johnsons – a father, mother, and their two children – started training as a way to spend quality time together. The dojo became their shared space, where they learned from each other and grew together, both as martial artists and as a family. Their story illustrates how Lightsaber MMA can strengthen family bonds, providing a unique and enjoyable way for families to connect and grow together.

The International Community:

In my travels, I've encountered the global community of Lightsaber MMA enthusiasts. This vibrant international network connects people from all corners of the world. Through forums, online training sessions, and international competitions, practitioners share techniques, experiences, and encouragement. It's a digital brotherhood and sisterhood that transcends geographical boundaries, showcasing the global reach and unifying power of Lightsaber MMA.

The personal anecdotes from the world of Lightsaber MMA are a testament to the powerful connections and friendships that can be formed through this unique discipline. Whether it's the bond between training partners, the mentorship between instructor and student, the unity among family members, or the camaraderie within the global community, Lightsaber MMA proves to be a catalyst for building meaningful, lasting relationships. It's more than a martial art; it's a journey of connection, unity, and shared human experience.

"The Power of Diversity in Martial Arts: A Community of Growth and Unity"

I have always believed in the power of community, especially one as diverse and engaging as that found in martial arts. Being part of such a community isn't just about learning self-defense or staying fit; it's a journey of personal growth, mutual respect, and global connection. Let's dive into the myriad benefits of immersing yourself in a diverse and engaging martial arts community.

Exposure to a Melting Pot of Cultures:
Martial arts communities are often vibrant tapestries of various cultures and backgrounds. By engaging in these communities, individuals gain a unique opportunity to interact with and learn from people from all walks of life. This exposure broadens perspectives, fosters cultural understanding, and nurtures an appreciation for diversity. It's a living example of how our differences make us stronger and more resilient.

Learning Beyond Techniques:
In a diverse martial arts community, learning goes beyond physical techniques. You're exposed to different philosophies, strategies,

and approaches to life. This diversity in learning styles and thought processes enhances cognitive flexibility, critical thinking, and problem-solving skills. It's a mental workout as much as it is physical, helping you grow in ways you might not have anticipated.

Building Respect and Empathy:

The martial arts ethos is deeply rooted in respect and empathy. In a diverse community, these values take on a deeper meaning. Practitioners learn to respect not just their teachers and the art but also the diverse backgrounds and experiences of their peers. This environment of mutual respect fosters empathy, understanding, and a sense of global citizenship.

Enhanced Communication and Social Skills:

Engaging with a diverse group of people in martial arts training hones communication and social skills. It teaches the art of listening, expressing oneself clearly, and the importance of non-verbal communication in understanding others. These skills are invaluable, transcending the dojo and impacting personal and professional life.

Fostering Teamwork and Leadership:

In a martial arts community, you often work in pairs or teams, learning to rely on and support each other. This dynamic enhances teamwork skills and can also foster leadership abilities. The diversity within the group means you encounter various team dynamics, preparing you for leadership roles in diverse settings.

Building Lifelong Friendships:

The bonds formed in martial arts communities often last a lifetime. These friendships are forged in the fires of shared challenges, victories, and growth. The diversity of the group adds richness to these relationships, offering a window into different life experiences and worldviews.

A Safe Space for Personal Growth:

A diverse and engaging martial arts community provides a safe space for personal growth. It's a place where you can challenge yourself, make mistakes, and learn in a supportive environment. The diversity of the group means you're exposed to various coping strategies and approaches to challenges, enriching your personal development journey.

Positive Impact on Mental Health:

Being part of a community, especially one as engaging and diverse as martial arts, has a positive impact on mental health. It combats feelings of loneliness and isolation, provides stress relief, and boosts self-esteem and confidence. The sense of belonging and being part of something larger than oneself is invaluable for emotional well-being.

Contributing to a Better World:

Finally, being part of a diverse martial arts community helps contribute to a more tolerant, understanding, and compassionate world. It teaches that despite our differences, we can come together, learn from each other, and grow together. Each individual, in their way, contributes to creating a global community rooted in respect, understanding, and unity.

The benefits of being part of a diverse and engaging martial arts community are profound and far-reaching. It's a journey that shapes not just your physical abilities but your character, worldview, and approach to life.

Participate in Lightsaber MMA groups and events to experience this community spirit.

CHAPTER FIVE

Common Misconceptions in Lightsaber MMA

Correcting Misunderstandings
  - Debunking the Novelty Myth
  - Correcting Misunderstandings About Practicality
  - Dispelling Myths About Accessibility and Inclusivity
  - The Misconception of Physical Intensity

Subsection: Correcting Misunderstandings

1. *Debunking the Novelty Myth*

A prevalent myth about Lightsaber MMA is that it's just a novelty, a temporary fad without any real depth. Let's dismantle this misconception. Lightsaber MMA is not merely a fleeting trend; it's a serious discipline that combines the physical rigor of martial arts with the strategic complexity of lightsaber combat.

"Unveiling the Depth of Lightsaber MMA: Beyond the Surface Appeal"

In my journeys, I've always been fascinated by disciplines that resonate deeply with people, inspiring them to discover more about themselves and their capabilities. Lightsaber Mixed Martial Arts (MMA) is one such discipline. At first glance, it might seem like a captivating blend of fantasy and sport, but as we delve deeper, we uncover a world rich in complexity, discipline, and transformative power.

A Fusion of Art and Science:

Lightsaber MMA is not just a physical activity; it's a confluence of art and science. The graceful movements, rooted in traditional martial arts, demand not only physical agility but also an understanding of biomechanics. Every strike, parry, and stance is a calculated expression of both power and poise, mirroring the dynamics of dance and combat. This fusion challenges practitioners to harmonize their mind and body, developing a heightened sense of awareness and control.

Cognitive and Emotional Development:

The training extends beyond the physical. Practitioners of Lightsaber MMA engage in a continuous process of cognitive and emotional growth. They learn to read their opponent's movements, anticipate actions, and make split-second decisions. This mental training sharpens their focus, enhances decision-making skills, and fosters a deep sense of mindfulness. Emotionally, it cultivates patience, resilience, and the ability to manage stress under pressure.

Philosophical and Ethical Underpinnings:

There is a profound philosophical and ethical dimension to Lightsaber MMA. Drawing from the rich lore of its sci-fi origins, it imparts lessons on morality, responsibility, and the balance between power and humility. Practitioners often find themselves reflecting on these themes, integrating them into their personal and professional lives. This philosophical depth encourages a holistic approach to life, emphasizing the importance of balance, integrity, and purpose.

Community and Leadership:

Beyond individual development, Lightsaber MMA fosters a strong sense of community and leadership. As practitioners advance, they often take on mentorship roles, guiding newer members. This transition from student to teacher reinforces leadership qualities like empathy, effective communication, and the ability to inspire and motivate others. The community itself becomes a space for sharing knowledge, celebrating diversity, and supporting collective growth.

Adaptability and Innovation:

The world of Lightsaber MMA is ever-evolving, encouraging constant adaptation and innovation. Practitioners are continually exploring new techniques, integrating technology, and pushing the boundaries of what is possible. This environment of continuous learning and adaptation is crucial in today's fast-paced, ever-changing world. It teaches the value of staying flexible, open-minded, and receptive to new ideas and approaches.

Physical and Mental Well-being:

The comprehensive training in Lightsaber MMA offers significant benefits for physical and mental well-being. Regular practice improves cardiovascular health, strength, flexibility, and overall physical fitness. Mentally, it provides a powerful outlet for stress relief, enhances self-esteem, and promotes a sense of inner peace and confidence.

Cultural Impact and Global Appeal:

Lightsaber MMA has a unique cultural impact, with its global appeal transcending language and cultural barriers. It unites people from different parts of the world, creating a shared language and experience. This universal appeal underscores the discipline's ability to bring people together, fostering understanding and collaboration across cultures.

Lightsaber MMA offers much more than its initial, captivating appeal. It is a discipline that encompasses physical fitness, cognitive skills, philosophical depth, community building, and cultural impact. It's complexity and transformative power make it not just a sport or hobby but a pathway to personal growth and global connection. As we engage with Lightsaber MMA, we discover a world where every swing of the saber is a step toward self-discovery, empowerment, and unity.

"Transformative Journeys: Personal Growth and Skill Mastery in Lightsaber MMA"

Over the years I've been privileged to witness numerous stories of transformation and growth. These stories aren't just about achieving goals; they're about profound personal journeys. Today, let's explore the inspiring stories of individuals who found not just skill development but deep personal growth through Lightsaber Mixed Martial Arts (MMA).

Tabitha's Journey from Doubt to Confidence:
Tabitha, a software engineer, initially saw Lightsaber MMA as a fun way to stay fit. What she didn't expect was how deeply it would impact her self-confidence. In the beginning, Tabitha struggled with self-doubt, often hesitating in her movements and decisions. Through persistent training, she not only honed her physical skills but also developed a new-found confidence that spilled over into her professional life. She learned to trust her instincts, make decisive moves, and embrace challenges, transforming not just as a martial artist but as a person.

David's Path to Mindfulness and Focus:
David, a busy executive, found in Lightsaber MMA an unexpected path to mindfulness. Juggling a demanding career and personal life,

he often felt scattered and stressed. The focused nature of Lightsaber training, however, taught him the art of mindfulness. Each session became a meditative practice, helping him to center his thoughts and be fully present. This new ability to focus and remain calm under pressure greatly improved his performance at work and his relationships at home.

Claudia's Story of Overcoming Fear:

For Claudia, a university student, Lightsaber MMA was a journey of overcoming fear. Having always been shy and reserved, stepping into the dojo was a challenge in itself. But as she engaged in the training, she began to confront and overcome her fears. Each strike and defense maneuver was a step out of her comfort zone, teaching her resilience and courage. Claudia's journey in Lightsaber MMA became a metaphor for life, showing her that she could face and conquer her fears.

Larry's Transition from Isolation to Community:

Larry, a freelance writer, initially took up Lightsaber MMA as a solitary pursuit. To his surprise, he found a vibrant community that welcomed him with open arms. This sense of belonging was new to Larry, who had often felt isolated in his work. The camaraderie and support he found in the dojo were transformative, providing him not just with friends but with a sense of being part of something greater than himself.

Anika's Integration of Discipline in Daily Life:

Anika, a young artist, was drawn to Lightsaber MMA for its aesthetic appeal but soon discovered the discipline it required. This discipline, which was initially challenging, gradually became a part of her daily life. The structure and dedication she practiced in her training began to influence her art and work ethic, leading to a more organized, purposeful approach to her career and creative projects.

Jordan's Breakthrough in Emotional Control:
For Jordan, a high school teacher, Lightsaber MMA became a tool for emotional control and release. Dealing with the daily stresses of teaching, he often found himself emotionally drained. Through Lightsaber MMA, he learned techniques to control and channel his emotions positively. The physical exertion was therapeutic, and the mental discipline it required helped him manage his emotions, leading to a more balanced and fulfilling life.

These stories from the Lightsaber MMA community remind us that the journey to mastery is about more than just developing physical skills. It's a transformative process that encompasses personal growth, mental fortitude, emotional control, and a deep connection with others. Each individual's story is a testament to the power of this practice in not just shaping the body but also molding the mind and spirit. As we listen to these tales, we are reminded of the limitless potential within each of us to grow, change, and become the best version of ourselves.

"Sustaining the Spark: Long-Term Benefits of Lightsaber MMA"

Often I've emphasized the importance of activities that not only ignite passion but also offer long-term benefits. Lightsaber Mixed Martial Arts (MMA) is a shining example of such an endeavor. It's not just a fleeting trend; it's a journey with lasting impacts. Let's explore the enduring benefits and sustained interest in Lightsaber MMA, and how it continues to enrich lives over time.

Continual Physical Development:
Lightsaber MMA is a dynamic sport that continuously challenges and develops the body. Unlike routines that might become monotonous over time, it offers endless opportunities for physical growth. Whether it's improving agility, strength, coordination, or endurance,

there's always a new level to strive for. This ongoing physical challenge keeps participants engaged and continuously progressing.

Mental Resilience and Adaptability:

The mental aspect of Lightsaber MMA cannot be overstated. Practitioners develop a resilience that transcends the dojo. They learn to adapt to new situations quickly, think on their feet, and remain calm under pressure. These skills are invaluable in everyday life, helping individuals to navigate personal and professional challenges with a clearer mind and a stronger sense of resolve.

Deepening Understanding of Martial Arts Principles:

As practitioners progress in Lightsaber MMA, their understanding of martial arts principles deepens. This discipline is rich in history and technique, offering a lifetime of learning. The more one delves into its intricacies, the more rewarding it becomes. This depth keeps practitioners engaged for years, as there is always more to explore and master.

Evolution of Personal Style and Technique:

Lightsaber MMA allows for the development of a personal style and technique. As individuals grow in the sport, they begin to tailor their approach to suit their strengths and preferences. This evolution is a deeply personal journey that keeps practitioners invested in their development, ensuring long-term engagement and interest.

Community and Social Connection:

The community aspect of Lightsaber MMA is a powerful factor in sustaining interest. Practitioners become part of a supportive and inspiring community. This social connection provides a sense of belonging and motivation to continue training. The relationships formed in this community often last a lifetime, providing continuous encouragement and camaraderie.

Holistic Health Benefits:

The holistic health benefits of Lightsaber MMA are a major factor in its long-term appeal. Regular practice promotes not just physical health but also mental and emotional well-being. The stress-relieving and mood-boosting effects of this discipline are profound, making it a valuable tool for maintaining overall health and happiness.

Personal Growth and Self-Discovery:

Finally, Lightsaber MMA is a journey of personal growth and self-discovery. As practitioners face and overcome challenges, they learn a lot about themselves. They develop confidence, self-discipline, and a sense of achievement that fuels their desire to continue. This personal growth is perhaps the most compelling reason why Lightsaber MMA holds such sustained interest.

Lightsaber MMA offers far more than just an initial thrill; it's a path to long-term development and fulfillment. Its blend of physical challenge, mental resilience, deep learning, community, and holistic health benefits ensures that it remains a captivating and enriching practice for years to come. For those seeking an activity that offers continuous growth and enduring interest, Lightsaber MMA is a journey worth embarking on.

Engage with long-term practitioners and attend advanced Lightsaber MMA sessions to see the depth firsthand.

2. Correcting Misunderstandings About Practicality

Another common misconception is that Lightsaber MMA isn't practical or applicable in real-world scenarios. However, the skills and techniques learned in Lightsaber MMA are about much more than handling a lightsaber; they enhance general combat skills, situational awareness, and physical fitness.

"Harnessing the Power of Lightsaber MMA for Real-Life Defense"

Often I stress the importance of skills that are not just transformative but also practical. One such remarkable area is Lightsaber Mixed Martial Arts (MMA) – a discipline that transcends the boundaries of traditional martial arts by integrating real-life self-defense and combat applications. Let's delve into how the unique blend of techniques and principles in Lightsaber MMA can be transferred to real-life situations, empowering individuals beyond the training arena.

Reflexes and Reaction Time:
At the heart of Lightsaber MMA training lies the development of quick reflexes and rapid reaction time. In real-world defense scenarios, the ability to respond swiftly and effectively can be lifesaving. The agility and speed honed in Lightsaber MMA directly translate to an enhanced ability to evade, block, and counter-attack in unforeseen circumstances. Practitioners find that their training in anticipating and reacting to moves provides them with a significant advantage in real-world situations.

Situational Awareness:
Lightsaber MMA teaches more than just physical skills; it instills a heightened sense of situational awareness. Practitioners learn to be acutely aware of their surroundings – a skill that is vital in identifying

potential threats in real life. This mindfulness, developed through focused training, enables individuals to navigate through various environments more securely and confidently.

Strategic Thinking and Decision Making:

In Lightsaber MMA, strategic thinking is crucial. Practitioners learn to assess their opponents, anticipate movements, and strategically plan their actions. This aspect of strategic thinking and rapid decision-making is invaluable in real-life self-defense situations, where assessing risks and making quick, informed decisions can make all the difference.

Emotional Control and Stress Management:

Combat situations, whether in the ring or on the streets, can be intense and emotionally taxing. Lightsaber MMA training includes managing stress and controlling emotions under pressure. This mental fortitude is crucial in real-life scenarios, where panic can be a formidable enemy. Practitioners learn to maintain composure, think clearly, and act decisively, even in the most stressful situations.

Endurance and Physical Toughness:

The rigorous physical training in Lightsaber MMA builds endurance and toughness, preparing individuals for the physical challenges of real-life combat. The conditioning exercises, sparring sessions, and endurance drills ensure that practitioners are not just skilled but also physically capable of defending themselves effectively.

Adaptability and Versatility:

Lightsaber MMA encompasses a wide range of techniques from various martial arts disciplines, making it a versatile and adaptable form of training. This diversity in skills ensures that practitioners are not limited to one style of fighting but are equipped with a comprehensive skill set that can be adapted to different real-life scenarios.

Empowerment and Confidence:

Beyond the physical and mental skills, Lightsaber MMA instills a deep sense of empowerment and confidence. Knowing that you possess the skills to defend yourself in adverse situations can be incredibly empowering. This confidence often translates to other areas of life, making individuals more assertive and proactive in their personal and professional endeavors.

Lightsaber MMA is a comprehensive training system that equips individuals with practical skills for real-life self-defense and combat situations. The lessons learned in the dojo go far beyond physical techniques, encompassing mental resilience, strategic thinking, and personal empowerment. For those seeking a martial art that offers real-world applicability, Lightsaber MMA stands out as a discipline that truly prepares its practitioners for the challenges they may face outside the training environment.

"From Dojo to Life: Real Stories of Lightsaber MMA in Action"

Today, I want to share with you inspiring stories from individuals who have taken their Lightsaber Mixed Martial Arts (MMA) training beyond the confines of a training facility and applied it in practical, real-world contexts. These anecdotes not only showcase the effectiveness of this unique martial art but also serve as a testament to the profound impact it can have on one's life.

Miley's Story: Confidence in Crisis:

Miley, a 28-year-old graphic designer, had always felt vulnerable walking home late at night. After a year of training in Lightsaber MMA, her perspective changed. One evening, she found herself in a potentially dangerous situation with a stranger following her. Drawing on her training, Miley maintained her composure, assessed her environment for escape routes, and prepared to defend herself if necessary.

Fortunately, the situation did not escalate, but Miley credits her Lightsaber MMA training for the confidence and alertness that empowered her during that tense moment.

Eugene's Turning Point: From Victim to Victor:
Eugene, a 35-year-old schoolteacher, had a harrowing experience of being mugged two years ago. This incident left him feeling helpless and anxious. Determined to regain his sense of control, Eugene took up Lightsaber MMA. Recently, when confronted by an aggressive individual, Eugene successfully de-escalated the situation using the verbal and non-verbal communication skills he learned in training. He credits Lightsaber MMA for transforming him from a victim to someone who can handle conflict assertively and peacefully.

Laura's Triumph: Overcoming Bullying:
High school can be challenging, and for 16-year-old Laura, it was a battleground due to bullying. After joining a Lightsaber MMA class, she found an outlet for her frustration and a boost in her self-esteem. The training gave her the courage to stand up for herself. She didn't have to fight; her newfound confidence and assertive body language were enough to deter the bullies and change her school life for the better.

Fred's Rescue: A Life Saved:
Fred, a 30-year-old nurse, found himself in a life-saving situation when a colleague collapsed from a heart attack. While others panicked, Fred's training in Lightsaber MMA had prepared him to stay calm under pressure. He administered CPR effectively until the paramedics arrived, a skill he perfected during his rigorous MMA training that emphasized precision and calmness under stress.

Jasmine's Journey: From Fear to Freedom:
Jasmine, a 40-year-old single mother, was once afraid to venture out into unfamiliar environments. After training in Lightsaber MMA, she

embarked on a solo hiking adventure, something she never thought possible. Her training taught her not just self-defense, but the importance of awareness, preparation, and self-reliance. She now travels regularly, exploring new places with confidence and enthusiasm.

These stories demonstrate that Lightsaber MMA is more than just a physical discipline; it is a transformative practice that equips individuals with the skills, confidence, and mental fortitude to face various challenges in life. Whether it's defending oneself in a dangerous situation, handling a conflict, overcoming personal hurdles, or even saving a life, the principles and techniques of Lightsaber MMA have proven their value in practical, real-world contexts. This martial art form does not just prepare you for combat; it prepares you for life, instilling in you the resilience, confidence, and adaptability needed to navigate the complexities of our modern world.

"Harnessing the Force of Full Preparedness: The Lightsaber MMA Way"

Let's delve into the remarkable world of Lightsaber Mixed Martial Arts (MMA) and its profound impact on both physical and mental preparedness. This unique blend of traditional martial arts and the iconic lightsaber not only revolutionizes physical fitness but also elevates mental fortitude to new heights.

1. Physical Preparedness – Beyond Traditional Boundaries:

Stamina and Strength:
Lightsaber MMA pushes the boundaries of physical endurance. Take the story of a 25-year-old aspiring athlete. He found his strength and stamina soaring as he mastered the lightsaber's

elegant movements. His journey in Lightsaber MMA transformed him from a casual gym-goer to an athlete with remarkable endurance.

Flexibility and Agility:

A 32-year-old yoga instructor, integrated Lightsaber MMA into her routine and noticed remarkable improvements in her flexibility and agility. The dynamic movements of Lightsaber MMA enhanced her body's fluidity, making her yoga practices more profound and effective.

Coordination and Balance:

For a 45-year-old accountant, the precision required in Lightsaber MMA drastically improved his coordination and balance. These skills have translated seamlessly into his daily life, making him more adept in his recreational sports and overall physical activities.

Self-Defense Skills:

A 29-year-old graphic designer, found confidence in her newfound self-defense abilities. Lightsaber MMA not only equipped her with practical defense techniques but also instilled a sense of empowerment that transcended the training dojo.

2. Mental Preparedness – A Journey to Inner Strength:

Focus and Concentration:

A 40-year-old entrepreneur, discovered that the concentration required in Lightsaber MMA dramatically improved his focus on business. This martial art demands a high level of attention to detail, which, when practiced regularly, spills over into every aspect of life.

Stress Relief and Mindfulness:

For a 35-year-old nurse, Lightsaber MMA became an outlet for stress relief. The immersive nature of the training allowed her to be present in the moment, offering a form of active mindfulness that was both exhilarating and calming.

Resilience and Perseverance:

A 22-year-old college student, faced numerous challenges both academically and personally. Through Lightsaber MMA, he learned the value of resilience. The discipline taught him that setbacks are not failures but opportunities for growth and learning.

Emotional Control and Self-Regulation:

A 28-year-old social worker found that Lightsaber MMA aided her in emotional regulation. The discipline required to master the art translated into better control over her emotions, helping her navigate the emotionally demanding aspects of her profession.

Lightsaber MMA is not just a sport or a hobby; it's a comprehensive training system that prepares individuals for the challenges of life. It strengthens the body, sharpens the mind, and enriches the spirit. Whether you are looking to improve your physical fitness, seeking mental clarity, or need a boost in your confidence, Lightsaber MMA offers a path to achieving these goals. It's a journey that prepares you for life's battles, teaches you the art of balance, and helps you discover your inner strength. Embrace the way of the Lightsaber, and you'll find yourself ready for anything life throws your way.

3. Dispelling Myths About Accessibility and Inclusivity

Some believe that Lightsaber MMA is exclusive and not welcoming to beginners or those outside the sci-fi fan base. This couldn't be further from the truth. Lightsaber MMA is an inclusive discipline, that welcomes individuals of all ages, backgrounds, and skill levels.

"Embracing Diversity in the Arena: The Inclusive World of Lightsaber MMA"

In the vast universe of martial arts, Lightsaber MMA stands out, not just for its unique blend of traditional discipline and modern flair, but for its remarkably inclusive training environments.

1. A Space for Everyone:

Breaking Barriers:
In the world of Lightsaber MMA, barriers of age, gender, and physical ability dissolve. Take Margret, a 50-year-old librarian, who discovered a new zest for life in her Lightsaber MMA class. Contrary to her initial apprehensions about her age, she found herself welcomed and empowered, training alongside teenagers and young adults.

Inclusivity for All Abilities:
Consider the story of Lawrence, a young man with a physical disability. Lightsaber MMA offered him an adaptable training program, where instructors tailored techniques to suit his capabilities. In this arena, his wheelchair became a part of his unique fighting style, not a limitation.

Gender Inclusivity:

Beth, a 30-year-old programmer, found in Lightsaber MMA a space free from gender stereotypes. In her dojo, women and men train together, learning from each other, and demonstrating that skill and passion transcend gender.

2. Cultivating Respect and Empathy:

Beyond Tolerance to Understanding:

Respect is a cornerstone in Lightsaber MMA. For instance, Paul, who comes from a different cultural background, found his classmates not only tolerant but genuinely interested in learning about his heritage. This mutual respect and curiosity create a rich learning environment.

Empathy in Action:

Training in Lightsaber MMA cultivates empathy. Natalie, a 25-year-old social worker, noticed how her ability to understand and connect with others improved, as the training emphasizes reading and responding to your opponent in a manner that respects their boundaries and abilities.

3. A Community of Support and Growth:

Bonding through Shared Passion:

The training sessions become more than just learning a skill; they are about building a community. Bart, a 40-year-old businessman, found a second family in his Lightsaber MMA class, where everyone supports each other's growth and celebrates their victories.

Personal Growth in a Safe Environment:

Lightsaber MMA offers a safe space for personal exploration. For someone like Lana, a shy 20-year-old student, the dojo became a place where she could express herself freely and build her confidence, surrounded by supportive peers and mentors.

4. Adaptable and Evolving:

Evolving with Times and Needs:

The art form is continually evolving, adapting to the needs of its diverse practitioners. Innovations in training techniques and equipment ensure that everyone, regardless of their physical condition or learning style, finds a place in Lightsaber MMA.

Global and Cultural Fusion:

Lightsaber MMA dojos often become melting pots of global cultures. Kevin, an immigrant, found a sense of belonging in a dojo that celebrated cultural diversity, integrating various martial arts styles from around the world.

Lightsaber MMA training environments are a testament to the power of inclusivity in sports. They prove that when we create spaces that welcome diversity, we enable individuals to not only learn a new skill but to embark on a transformative journey of personal growth, mutual respect, and community building. In the dojo of Lightsaber MMA, every individual, regardless of their background, is not just accepted but celebrated.

Visit a Lightsaber MMA class or workshop to experience this welcoming atmosphere.

4. The Misconception of Physical Intensity

A misconception exists that Lightsaber MMA is overly intense and physically demanding, suitable only for those at peak fitness levels. In reality, Lightsaber MMA caters to a wide range of physical abilities, offering scalable challenges suitable for everyone.

"Adaptable Training, Universal Wellness: The Role of Lightsaber MMA for All Fitness Levels"

Let's take a moment to delve into the adaptable nature of Lightsaber MMA training and its role in enhancing physical health and wellness for practitioners across various fitness levels. Lightsaber MMA is not just a sport; it's a pathway to holistic wellness, tailored to meet the unique needs and capabilities of each individual.

1. Adaptability for All Fitness Levels:

Personalized Training Approaches:
Envision a training environment where each session is customized to meet the individual needs of the students. For beginners, the pace is gentle and progressively intensifies, allowing gradual improvement in fitness and skill.

Inclusive Techniques for Varied Abilities:
Instructors often develop modified techniques to accommodate individuals with physical limitations, ensuring everyone can participate fully and safely, irrespective of their physical challenges.

2. Promoting Physical Health:

Comprehensive Fitness Development:

Participants from various walks of life experience improvements in strength, endurance, and flexibility, highlighting the sport's well-rounded approach to physical health.

Safe and Effective Exercise Regimen:

For those seeking a blend of cardio, strength training, and agility exercises, Lightsaber MMA offers a comprehensive and structured environment, emphasizing its effectiveness as an all-encompassing exercise regimen.

3. Wellness for All Practitioners:

Mental and Physical Symbiosis:

The mental focus required in Lightsaber MMA complements the physical exertion, leading to improved overall wellness, especially beneficial for those dealing with stress or mental fatigue.

Adaptation to Lifestyle Changes:

The sport adapts to the changing lifestyles of its practitioners, offering less intensive but equally engaging routines for those in different life stages, including the elderly or those with reduced mobility.

4. Long-term Health Benefits:

Sustained Physical Activity:
The evolving nature of Lightsaber MMA keeps practitioners consistently engaged, ensuring ongoing physical activity and long-term health benefits.

Holistic Health Approach:
The training emphasizes not just physical health but also incorporates breathing techniques and mindfulness, promoting a holistic approach to wellness.

Lightsaber MMA stands as a model of adaptable training, welcoming everyone from novices to advanced athletes, young and old alike. Its comprehensive training underlines the importance of physical health, while its adaptable nature ensures that everyone, regardless of fitness level or physical constraints, can reap its benefits. Lightsaber MMA transcends the realm of sport, emerging as a portal to a healthier, more active lifestyle, fostering both physical and mental wellness. Let's embrace this adaptable, inclusive martial art and unlock our potential for comprehensive wellness.

CHAPTER SIX

Secrets to Mastery:

Advanced Lightsaber MMA Techniques

Exploring Advanced Techniques and Strategies
- The Art of Lightsaber Combat
- Developing Strategic Mindset in Combat
- Holistic Training for Physical and Mental Agility
- The Role of Emotional Intelligence in Mastery

Subsection: Exploring Advanced Techniques and Strategies

1. *The Art of Lightsaber Combat*

Mastery in Lightsaber MMA goes beyond basic combat; it involves mastering an art form. This segment of the journey is where technique meets creativity, and strategy intertwines with physical prowess.

"Adaptable Training, Universal Wellness: The Role of Lightsaber MMA for All Fitness Levels"

Lightsaber MMA is not just a sport; it's a pathway to holistic wellness, tailored to meet the unique needs and capabilities of each individual.

1. Adaptability for All Fitness Levels:

Personalized Training Approaches:
Envision a training environment where each session is customized to meet the individual needs of the students. For beginners, the pace is gentle and progressively intensifies, allowing gradual improvement in fitness and skill.

Inclusive Techniques for Varied Abilities:
Instructors often develop modified techniques to accommodate individuals with physical limitations, ensuring everyone can participate fully and safely, irrespective of their physical challenges.

2. Promoting Physical Health:

Comprehensive Fitness Development:
Participants from various walks of life experience improvements in strength, endurance, and flexibility, highlighting the sport's well-rounded approach to physical health.

Safe and Effective Exercise Regimen:
For those seeking a blend of cardio, strength training, and agility exercises, Lightsaber MMA

offers a comprehensive and structured environment, emphasizing its effectiveness as an all-encompassing exercise regimen.

3. Wellness for All Practitioners:

Mental and Physical Symbiosis:

The mental focus required in Lightsaber MMA complements the physical exertion, leading to improved overall wellness, especially beneficial for those dealing with stress or mental fatigue.

Adaptation to Lifestyle Changes:

The sport adapts to the changing lifestyles of its practitioners, offering less intensive but equally engaging routines for those in different life stages, including the elderly or those with reduced mobility.

4. Long-term Health Benefits:

Sustained Physical Activity:

The evolving nature of Lightsaber MMA keeps practitioners consistently engaged, ensuring ongoing physical activity and long-term health benefits.

Holistic Health Approach:

The training emphasizes not just physical health but also incorporates breathing techniques and mindfulness, promoting a holistic approach to wellness.

Lightsaber MMA stands as a model of adaptable training, welcoming everyone from novices to advanced athletes, young and old alike. Its comprehensive training underlines the importance of physical health, while its adaptable nature ensures that everyone, regardless of fitness level or physical constraints, can reap its benefits. Lightsaber MMA transcends the realm of sport, emerging as a portal to a healthier, more active lifestyle, fostering both physical and mental wellness. Let's embrace this adaptable, inclusive martial art and unlock our potential for comprehensive wellness.

"Mastering the Blade: How Advanced Lightsaber Combat Skills Enhance Reflexes and Strategic Thinking"

The world of advanced lightsaber combat skills is not just a flashy sport; it's a discipline that sharpens your reflexes and hones your strategic thinking. Let's explore how mastering these skills can transform you, not just as a martial artist, but as an individual.

1. Enhanced Reflexes - The Quickening of Body and Mind:

Instantaneous Response: In the heat of lightsaber combat, there's no time for hesitation. Every attack and defense requires instantaneous reflexes. As you train, your body learns to react faster, almost with a mind of its own. This quickening isn't just physical – it's a mental sharpening, a readiness that spills over into every aspect of life.

Anticipation and Adaptation: With each spar, you learn to anticipate your opponent's moves. This foresight isn't just about seeing; it's about feeling the rhythm of the battle. It's about adapting to the unexpected, a skill that is invaluable in both personal and professional realms.

2. Strategic Thinking - Beyond the Duel:

The Art of Strategy: Lightsaber combat is like a high-speed game of chess. Every move has a purpose, every decision has consequences. Advanced training teaches you to think several steps ahead, to strategize not just for the immediate, but for the endgame.

Mental Agility: This form of combat encourages mental agility. You learn to quickly assess situations, to pivot strategies on the fly. This agility is a powerful tool. It sharpens your decision-making skills, enabling you to navigate complex situations with ease.

3. From Combat to Daily Life - Transferring Skills:

Application in Everyday Life: The reflexes and strategic thinking developed in lightsaber combat have real-world applications. Whether it's making quick decisions in a business meeting or reacting to unexpected life events, these skills empower you to act with confidence and clarity.

Continuous Improvement: Advanced lightsaber training is a journey of continuous improvement. It's about challenging yourself and pushing beyond your limits. It instills a growth mindset, a belief that with persistence and practice, you can excel.

4. The Bigger Picture - Personal and Professional Growth:

Confidence and Presence: As your skills grow, so does your confidence. There's a sense of presence, a composure that comes with knowing you can handle high-pressure situations. This confidence radiates, affecting every interaction in, every relationship.

Leadership and Teamwork: In advanced training, you often work in teams. This fosters leadership skills and a deep sense of teamwork and collaboration. These are qualities that define great leaders in any field.

Advanced lightsaber combat training offers much more than physical prowess. It shapes your reflexes, making them razor-sharp. It molds your mind, teaching you the art of strategy and anticipation. These skills transfer seamlessly into everyday life, enhancing your personal and professional development. As you master the blade, you also master aspects of yourself, unlocking potentials you never knew existed. Remember, the path of mastery is endless, but every step on this path is a step towards a more empowered, more resilient you. So, embrace the journey, and let the force of your determination guide you.

2. Developing Strategic Mindset in Combat

In Lightsaber MMA, physical skill is just one part of the equation. Developing a strategic mindset is crucial for anticipating opponents' moves and planning your strategy in real time.

"The Mind-Blade Connection: Mental Agility and Strategic Planning in Lightsaber MMA"

Lightsaber MMA. It's more than just a physical challenge; it's a mental game that requires agility and strategic foresight. Let's dive into how mental agility and strategic planning are crucial in mastering Lightsaber MMA.

1. Mental Agility: The Heart of Combat:

Split-Second Decision Making: In Lightsaber MMA, every moment is unpredictable. Mental agility is the ability to make quick, effective decisions. It's about processing information rapidly and responding with precision. This skill is vital not only in combat but in every facet of life, where quick decision-making can mean the difference between success and failure.

Adaptability in Action: Agility means adaptability. In the throes of a duel, no plan survives first contact unchanged. Being mentally agile allows you to adapt your strategy on the fly, to turn setbacks into opportunities. This adaptability is a life skill, which teaches you to remain flexible and resilient in the face of change.

2. Strategic Planning: The Blueprint of Success:

The Art of Prediction: Strategic planning in Lightsaber MMA is about predicting your opponent's moves and preparing countermeasures. It's a deep understanding of both your and your opponent's strengths and weaknesses.

This level of foresight is crucial in life, where anticipating challenges can help you navigate them more effectively.

Long-Term Vision: A good strategy in Lightsaber MMA is not just about the immediate duel; it's about the long-term development of your skills. It's about setting goals and crafting a pathway to achieve them. This long-term vision is essential in personal and professional growth, helping you to set and achieve meaningful objectives.

3. Combining Agility with Strategy:

Dynamic Balance: The true mastery of Lightsaber MMA lies in balancing mental agility with strategic planning. It's about being flexible while staying true to your plan. This dynamic balance is key in life, where being rigid can lead to failure, and being too impulsive can lead to recklessness.

Continuous Learning and Growth: Lightsaber MMA is a journey of continuous learning. Each duel is a lesson, and each practice session is a chance to grow. This mindset of continuous improvement is invaluable, encouraging you to always seek personal and professional development.

4. Application Beyond the Arena:

Everyday Life Skills: The mental skills developed in Lightsaber MMA are transferable to everyday life. Mental agility helps you navigate complex situations at work or home. Strategic planning assists in making life decisions that align with your long-term goals.

Enhanced Professional Abilities: In the professional world, these skills enhance your ability to lead, innovate, and solve problems. Whether you're an entrepreneur, a teacher, or an artist, the mental agility and strategic planning honed in Lightsaber MMA can elevate your professional capabilities.

Lightsaber MMA is not just about physical strength and skill. It's a discipline that sharpens your mind, teaching you the art of mental agility and strategic planning. These skills are invaluable, enhancing your ability to make decisions, adapt to change, and plan for success in all areas of life.

"Mastering the Art of Strategy: Tales from the Lightsaber Arena"

The electrifying world of lightsaber combat, a realm where strategy isn't just a part of the game – it is the game. Let me share with you some inspiring stories that highlight the power of strategy in this dynamic sport.

The Underdog's Triumph:
Imagine a scenario where an inexperienced contender faces a seasoned champion. The odds are stacked against the newcomer, but what they lack in experience, they make up for in strategic planning. They study their opponent, learning their patterns and weaknesses. In the arena, they use feints and unpredictable maneuvers, turning the tide. This underdog's victory isn't just a win; it's a testament to the power of strategic thinking, proving that with the right plan, even giants can be toppled.

The Duel of Wits:

Picture a duel that seemed evenly matched, with two combatants mirroring each other's every move. But as the bout progresses, one of them begins to take a slight lead, not through physical superiority but through superior strategy. They start varying their attack patterns, keeping their opponent guessing. This psychological warfare drains the opponent's mental energy, leading to a small but crucial mistake – and that's all it takes. This story illustrates that lightsaber combat is as much a duel of wits as it is of blades.

The Team Tactic:

Let's shift focus to a team scenario. A group of practitioners, diverse in their styles, come together for a tournament. Initially, their different approaches seem to clash, but soon they realize the power of combining their unique strategies. They develop a plan that utilizes each member's strengths and covers their weaknesses. This unified approach leads them to victory against teams that might be individually stronger but lack a cohesive strategy. This narrative highlights the importance of adaptability and teamwork in strategic planning.

The Veteran's Adaptation:

Consider a veteran of the sport, known for their traditional approach. Over time, they notice the evolving nature of the game, with new techniques emerging. Instead of resisting change, they embrace it, integrating new strategies into their repertoire. This adaptability revitalizes their career, allowing them to compete with newer, younger contenders. It's a powerful reminder that in lightsaber combat, and life, being open to new strategies is key to sustained success.

The Comeback Story:

Finally, think of a combatant who suffers a major defeat. Instead of being disheartened, they use this as a learning opportunity. They analyze their performance, identifying strategic errors and areas for improvement. They train with a renewed focus on strategy, not just skill. In their next encounter, they emerge victorious, a clear indication of how critical strategic planning and learning from failures is to mastering lightsaber combat.

In conclusion, these stories from the lightsaber arena demonstrate the undeniable importance of strategy in achieving success. They show that while physical skill is important, it's the mind that ultimately leads to victory. Whether you're an underdog, a veteran, part of a team, or on a journey of a comeback, remember: in lightsaber combat, as in life, a well-crafted strategy can be your most powerful weapon. Keep these tales in mind as you forge your path, and let the art of strategy guide you to your victories.

"The Mental Edge: Strategic Combat's Role in Sharpening the Mind"

Disciplines like Lightsaber MMA, enhance mental acuity and decision-making skills. This fascinating journey is a cerebral voyage that fine-tunes the mind.

The Arena of Strategic Thinking:

Strategic combat isn't merely a test of physical strength; it's a chess game in motion. Each move, each decision, is a question posed to the opponent. Practitioners must think several steps ahead, anticipating and countering their opponent's strategies. This constant mental engagement sharpens the brain, improving problem-solving skills and strategic thinking.

Decisiveness in the Face of Adversity:

In the heat of combat, there's little room for hesitation. Practitioners must make split-second decisions, often under intense pressure. This environment fosters decisiveness, an invaluable skill in and out of the arena. It's about assessing the situation rapidly, weighing options, and committing to a course of action with confidence.

Adaptability: The Mental Flexibility:

Strategic combat is unpredictable. Opponents may change tactics, or unforeseen situations may arise. This unpredictability teaches mental adaptability – the ability to change strategies on the fly. Such mental agility is crucial in today's fast-paced world, where flexibility and adaptability are keys to success in personal and professional spheres.

Concentration and Focus:

Engaging in strategic combat requires intense concentration. Practitioners must focus on their opponent, anticipate moves, and be aware of their surroundings. This level of focus enhances the ability to concentrate, a skill that translates into improved attention and mindfulness in other areas of life.

The Resilience Factor:

Strategic combat is as much about mental resilience as it is about physical endurance. Facing challenges and overcoming setbacks in the arena builds mental toughness. This resilience is a cornerstone of mental acuity, as it fosters a mindset that sees challenges as opportunities for growth rather than insurmountable obstacles.

Learning from Failure:

In strategic combat, every misstep is a learning opportunity. Practitioners analyze their defeats, understand their mistakes, and devise new strategies. This process enhances critical thinking and learning from failure – essential components of effective decision-making.

Empathy and Understanding the Opponent:

To outmaneuver an opponent, one must understand them. Strategic combatants often learn to read body language, predict patterns, and understand their opponent's mindset. This fosters a kind of empathetic intelligence, allowing for better understanding and prediction of others' actions, a vital skill in all interpersonal interactions.

The Zen of Strategy:

Lastly, strategic combat often involves a state of flow, a mental state where a person is fully immersed in an activity. Achieving this state through combat practice can lead to greater mental clarity, reduced stress, and an overall sense of well-being.

The benefits of strategic combat extend far beyond the physical. It molds the mind, enhancing mental acuity, decision-making skills, focus, adaptability, and resilience. Whether in a lightsaber duel or the challenges of daily life, the mental skills honed in the arena are invaluable assets, helping practitioners navigate life with a sharper, more strategic mind. In the art of strategic combat, every move is a lesson, not just in physicality, but in the power of the human mind.

3. Holistic Training for Physical and Mental Agility

Achieving mastery in Lightsaber MMA requires a holistic approach to training, focusing on both physical agility and mental acuity.

"The Synchronized Dance of Mind and Body: Achieving Agility and Quickness"

The essential balance of physical training and mental exercises is to achieve not just physical agility but mental quickness as well.

The Fusion of Physical and Mental Training:
Physical training in disciplines like Lightsaber MMA is a given. It demands agility, strength, and endurance. However, the secret sauce to truly excelling in any physical discipline lies in the harmonious balance with mental training. It's about uniting the agility of the body with the quickness of the mind.

Physical Training: More Than Just Muscle:
Physical exercises do more than build muscle; they enhance neuroplasticity. Every physical movement refines our motor skills, fine-tunes our reflexes, and improves our neural efficiency. Techniques practiced in disciplines like Lightsaber MMA not only hone the body's agility but also train the brain to process information faster and respond in a fraction of a second.

Mental Exercises: Sharpening the Mind:
The mind is the ultimate tool in any combat art. Mental exercises such as visualization, strategic games, and meditation are integral. They sharpen focus, enhance decision-making skills, and cultivate a mindset that anticipates and outmaneuvers the opponent. This mental agility allows for quicker adaptation and response in high-pressure situations.

The Power of Visualization:

Visualization is a potent tool. It involves mentally rehearsing movements and scenarios, creating neural pathways similar to those formed during actual physical practice. This mental rehearsal not only prepares the mind but also enhances muscle memory, allowing for quicker, more fluid physical responses.

Strategic Games: Training the Tactical Mind:

Engaging in strategic games like chess or even certain video games can significantly improve tactical thinking. These activities sharpen the mind, enhance problem-solving skills, and teach the art of anticipation. They mirror the strategic planning required in physical combat, improving overall mental acuity.

Meditation: The Focus Catalyst:

Meditation isn't just for relaxation; it's a crucial training tool for the mind. It enhances concentration, calms the mind, and reduces reaction time. A calm, focused mind can better navigate the chaos of physical combat, making decisions with clarity and rapidity.

Physical and Mental Synergy in Practice:

A balanced training regime combines physical drills with mental exercises. For instance, a Lightsaber MMA practitioner might follow a physical workout with a meditation session or engage in visualization techniques before a sparring match. This synergy ensures that both mind and body react as one cohesive unit.

Adapting Training to Individual Needs:

Everyone's journey to achieving agility and quickness is unique. Some may require more focus on mental training, while others may need to enhance their physical regimen. The key is to identify personal areas of improvement and tailor a balanced training approach that addresses both physical and mental aspects.

The End Goal: Total Agility:
The goal isn't just to be physically quick or mentally sharp; it's to achieve total agility. Total agility means being able to think on your feet, adapt to new challenges instantly, and move with precision and purpose. It's about being prepared for anything life throws at you, both inside and outside the arena.

Mastering a discipline like a Lightsaber MMA goes beyond physical prowess. It's about nurturing a quick, strategic mind in tandem with a nimble, agile body. By balancing physical training with mental exercises, practitioners can achieve a level of overall agility and quickness that transcends the bounds of the training ground and permeates every aspect of life.

"Integrating Lightsabers in Mind-Body Mastery: Innovative Training Routines"

Let's dive into how lightsabers can be creatively incorporated into training routines that challenge both the mind and body, elevating the practice of lightsaber martial arts to new heights.

1. Lightsaber Drills with Memory Enhancement:
Imagine practicing swift lightsaber sequences, each move flowing into the next. While executing these sequences, participants also engage in memory exercises, like reciting sequences of numbers or strategic game moves. This combination sharpens reflexes and memory, fostering a sharper mind and a more agile body.

2. Strategic Lightsaber Sparring:
Sparring with lightsabers isn't just a physical endeavor; it's a mental chess game. Practitioners can be assigned specific strategic

objectives during sparring, such as disarming an opponent using a limited set of moves. This routine cultivates strategic thinking alongside physical prowess.

3. Visualization-Reaction Drills with Lightsabers:

Participants close their eyes and visualize an opponent's attack. Upon a signal, they instantly react, lightsaber in hand, executing a precise defensive or offensive maneuver. This enhances mental readiness and improves reaction times, essential for lightsaber combat.

4. Lightsaber Obstacle Courses:

Create an obstacle course where each station involves a unique challenge combining lightsaber skills with problem-solving. Navigating these courses under time pressure hones decision-making skills and physical agility, integral to lightsaber martial arts.

5. Balancing Acts with Cognitive Tasks:

Balancing on a beam while wielding a lightsaber, participants solve math problems or respond to trivia. The focus required to maintain balance with the lightsaber, coupled with the mental effort to solve problems, trains the brain and body simultaneously.

6. Endurance Training with Tactical Planning:

Imagine long-distance runs or cycling sessions where practitioners carry lightsabers. During this, they mentally map out battle strategies or plan complex lightsaber forms. This endurance training builds stamina while sharpening the tactical mind.

7. Lightsaber Forms with Cognitive Sequencing:

Executing intricate lightsaber forms while simultaneously recalling and implementing complex tactical sequences enhances cognitive abilities. This practice not only perfects the art of lightsaber combat but also strengthens mental discipline and strategic thinking.

8. Interactive Dueling Scenarios:
Participants engage in scenario-based duels where each encounter is designed with specific challenges and storylines. These scenarios require quick thinking, adaptability, and mastery of lightsaber techniques, providing a holistic training experience.

Incorporating lightsabers into these routines isn't just about physical training; it's about creating a harmonious synergy between the mind and body, essential for mastering the art of lightsaber combat. By challenging both aspects simultaneously, practitioners develop a deeper, more profound understanding of this unique martial art.

"Harnessing Holistic Training for Mastery in Lightsaber MMA"

In the realm of Lightsaber MMA, the quest for excellence transcends mere physical prowess. It's a journey that demands the integration of mind, body, and spirit - a holistic approach that is not just beneficial but essential for peak performance. Here's why:

Mind-Body Synchronization:
In Lightsaber MMA, every move is a dance of precision and grace. A holistic training approach emphasizes the synchronization of mental focus with physical agility. Through meditative practices coupled with rigorous physical drills, practitioners develop an acute awareness of their bodies, enhancing coordination and fluidity in their movements. This synergy is the cornerstone of mastering complex lightsaber forms and techniques.

Enhanced Mental Resilience:

The mental aspect of Lightsaber MMA cannot be overstated. Holistic training includes cognitive exercises that sharpen focus, boost strategic thinking, and foster quick decision-making under pressure. Techniques like visualization and mindfulness not only hone mental acuity but also build resilience, enabling practitioners to remain calm and collected in the face of intense competition.

Emotional Balance and Control:

The emotional landscape of a lightsaber duel is as varied and tumultuous as the physical one. A holistic approach teaches practitioners to channel their emotions, transforming fear and aggression into passion and drive. Emotional control is critical in maintaining composure during a duel, allowing one to respond rather than react.

Physical Conditioning and Agility:

While Lightsaber MMA is an art, it is also an intense physical activity that demands strength, endurance, and flexibility. Holistic training goes beyond basic fitness; it incorporates a range of activities like yoga, Pilates, and dynamic stretching. This not only improves overall physical health but also prevents injuries, ensuring a longer, healthier practice.

Spiritual Growth and Connection:

At its heart, Lightsaber MMA is more than a sport; it's a spiritual journey. The holistic approach fosters a deep connection with oneself and the larger community. It's about respecting the art, understanding its history, and appreciating its philosophy. This spiritual aspect adds depth to the practice, enriching the experience beyond the physical realm.

Nutritional Awareness:

A warrior's body is their temple, and how they fuel it is crucial. Holistic training emphasizes the importance of nutrition in performance. Tailored dietary plans that cater to the unique needs of each practitioner ensure optimal energy levels and recovery, essential for the rigors of Lightsaber MMA.

Rest and Recovery:

In the relentless pursuit of excellence, rest can often be overlooked. However, holistic training understands that recovery is as vital as practice. Techniques like sleep optimization, relaxation exercises, and restorative practices are integral, allowing the body and mind to recuperate and grow stronger.

Community and Support:

Lastly, the holistic approach is about being part of a community. Lightsaber MMA is not a solitary journey; it thrives on the support, shared knowledge, and camaraderie of fellow practitioners. This sense of belonging not only motivates but also provides a valuable network for learning and growth.

A holistic training approach in Lightsaber MMA is the key to unlocking one's full potential. It fully nurtures the practitioner, addressing every aspect that contributes to their overall performance. This approach doesn't just create skilled fighters; it molds well-rounded individuals who excel in every aspect of life.

4. The Role of Emotional Intelligence in Mastery

Emotional intelligence plays a pivotal role in mastering Lightsaber MMA. Controlling emotions under pressure and reading opponents' emotional cues are skills that separate good practitioners from true masters.

"Mastering Emotional Control and Awareness in Combat Situations"

Let's understand the critical impact of emotional control and awareness in combat situations, particularly in the dynamic world of Lightsaber MMA.

When we talk about combat, whether in martial arts or life's many battles, mastering emotional control and awareness is not just beneficial – it's vital. Here's why:

Emotional Control – The Key to Clarity:
In the heat of combat, emotions can run high. Fear, anger, excitement – all these feelings can cloud judgment and lead to impulsive decisions. Emotional control is about maintaining clarity and focus, ensuring that each move is calculated and deliberate. In Lightsaber MMA, this means being able to read your opponent, anticipate their next move, and strategically plan your response, rather than reacting out of fear or aggression.

Understanding the 'Fight or Flight' Response:
Our natural 'fight or flight' response can be both a friend and a foe. Awareness of this instinctual reaction allows combatants to channel adrenaline positively, using it to enhance performance rather than becoming paralyzed by it. This awareness is crucial in Lightsaber MMA, where split-second decisions can mean the difference between victory and defeat.

The Role of Emotional Intelligence:
Emotional intelligence is a powerful tool in combat. It involves not only managing your own emotions but also reading and responding to those of your opponent. In Lightsaber MMA, understanding your opponent's emotional state can provide valuable insights into their next move, enabling you to counteract effectively.

Stress Management Techniques:
Combat situations, especially in competitive settings like Lightsaber MMA, can be incredibly stressful. Employing stress management techniques like deep breathing, mindfulness, and visualization can help maintain emotional equilibrium, keeping you calm and focused under pressure.

Building Mental Resilience:
Emotional control contributes to mental resilience, a trait that is invaluable in combat sports. Mental resilience helps you bounce back from setbacks, remain undeterred by fear, and stay committed to your strategy, even when things don't go as planned.

Training for Emotional Endurance:

Just as physical endurance is built through training, so is emotional endurance. Regular practice under stressful conditions, such as high-intensity sparring sessions, can condition the mind to handle the emotional pressures of real combat. This training is essential in Lightsaber MMA, where the mental game is as important as the physical one.

The Power of Positive Affirmations:

Positive affirmations can reinforce emotional control. Reminding yourself of your strengths, abilities, and strategy can boost confidence, reduce anxiety, and keep you centered. In Lightsaber MMA, this could mean reciting a personal mantra before stepping into the ring, ensuring that you're mentally prepared for the challenge ahead.

The Role of a Supportive Community:

Finally, a supportive community plays a vital role in developing emotional control. In Lightsaber MMA, training with a team that understands and supports your emotional journey can provide a safe space to explore and master your emotions, leading to better performance in combat situations.

Emotional control and awareness are indispensable tools in any combat situation. In the world of Lightsaber MMA, where the blend of physical skill and mental strategy defines success, mastering these aspects can elevate a practitioner from a mere competitor to a true warrior. In the arena of combat, the most powerful weapon is not the lightsaber, but the mind that wields it.

"Harnessing Emotional Intelligence in Lightsaber Duels"

I want to share with you some powerful anecdotes that demonstrate the incredible effectiveness of emotional intelligence in lightsaber duels. Lightsaber duels are not just a test of physical prowess, but also a profound display of mental strength and emotional control.

1. The Duel of Anticipation:

In a recent lightsaber competition, two formidable opponents faced off. One was known for their technical skill, the other for their ability to read opponents. As the duel commenced, it was evident that the latter was using emotional intelligence to anticipate moves. By reading subtle body language cues and understanding the emotional mindset of their opponent, they were able to predict and counter moves with astonishing accuracy. This duel was not won by physical strength but by the power of understanding and anticipation.

2. The Power of Calmness:

Another practitioner, during an intense sparring session, was known for their fiery temperament. However, they learned to harness the power of calmness, a vital aspect of emotional intelligence. Through deep breathing and self-awareness exercises, they transformed their combat style. Instead of reacting impulsively, they began to respond with thoughtfulness and precision, turning their previous weakness into a formidable strength.

3. Overcoming Fear:

A young duelist once shared with me their struggle with fear and self-doubt. These emotions would cloud their judgment during duels. Through emotional intelligence training, they learned to recognize and understand these emotions without letting them take control. This newfound awareness led to a significant improvement in their performance, as they could now duel with confidence and clear focus.

4. The Empathetic Duelist:

In a championship, a competitor was known for their empathetic approach. They could sense the frustration and impatience in their opponents and would use this insight to their advantage. By staying one step ahead emotionally, they were able to wear down their opponents, proving that empathy can be a powerful tool in combat.

5. The Art of Self-Control:

During an intense match, one participant displayed exceptional self-control. Despite provocations and attempts to unbalance them emotionally, they remained centered and focused. This emotional stability allowed them to maintain a clear strategy and eventually win the duel, showcasing the importance of self-control in high-pressure situations.

6. Emotional Resilience in Defeat:

Emotional intelligence is not just about how one handles victory, but also defeat. A seasoned duelist once shared how they use losses as opportunities for growth. By handling defeat with grace and analyzing their emotional responses, they learned valuable lessons that improved their future performances.

These lightsaber duels illustrate the profound impact emotional intelligence has on performance. It's not just about the physical skills, but also about understanding and controlling your emotions, empathizing with your opponent, and using this awareness to make strategic decisions. Remember, in the realm of lightsaber duels, and indeed in all aspects of life, mastering emotional intelligence can be your greatest asset. Embrace it, and watch as it transforms not just your combat skills, but your entire approach to challenges.

"Emotional Intelligence: The Key to Resilience and Adaptability in Lightsaber MMA"

Mastering emotional intelligence contributes to resilience and adaptability in the exhilarating world of Lightsaber MMA. This unique martial art is more than just physical agility; it's a journey towards emotional mastery.

Emotional Awareness and Resilience:
In Lightsaber MMA, understanding your emotions is crucial. Picture a scenario where a duelist faces an unexpected setback. Instead of succumbing to frustration, those with high emotional intelligence recognize and regulate their feelings. They use this awareness to stay composed, bounce back quickly, and adapt their strategy. This emotional resilience is vital, transforming potential defeat into a learning experience that strengthens their resolve.

Empathy and Tactical Advantage:
Empathy, a core component of emotional intelligence, is about understanding others' emotions. In a duel, perceiving an opponent's emotional state – be it overconfidence or hesitation – provides a tactical edge. Duelists with high emotional intelligence read these cues and adjust their approach, often outmaneuvering their opponents not by physical force, but by strategic thinking.

Self-Regulation and Consistency:
Self-regulation in Lightsaber MMA is about maintaining control over one's emotions, especially under pressure. This aspect of emotional intelligence ensures a consistent performance regardless of the situation. A duelist might face intense pressure or provocation, but by mastering self-regulation, they remain

focused, making decisions that are strategic and calculated rather than reactive.

The Role of Emotional Agility:

Emotional agility is the ability to manage one's thoughts and feelings in diverse and challenging situations. Imagine a duelist navigating through a high-stakes tournament. The journey is filled with ups and downs, intense pressure, and fierce competition. Emotional agility enables them to remain flexible, adapt to changing circumstances, and pivot strategies as needed, all while keeping their emotions in check.

Social Awareness and Community Building:

Lightsaber MMA is not just an individual pursuit; it's a community. Emotional intelligence fosters a sense of belonging and camaraderie. Duelists with high social awareness build strong relationships, offer support, and create an environment where everyone feels valued. This sense of community is vital for personal growth and the collective advancement of the art.

Emotional Intelligence in Training:

The training for Lightsaber MMA is rigorous, both physically and mentally. Emotional intelligence plays a crucial role here as well. It enables practitioners to approach their training with discipline and a positive mindset, to accept feedback constructively, and to set realistic goals. This approach enhances the overall training experience, leading to continuous improvement.

Emotional intelligence is a cornerstone of excellence in Lightsaber MMA. It's about more than just understanding and managing your emotions; it's about using this understanding to become more resilient, adaptable, and tactically sound. It's about building meaningful connections and nurturing a supportive community. As you embark on your Lightsaber MMA journey, remember that the path to mastery involves not just physical training but also the development of your emotional intelligence.

Practice mindfulness and emotional awareness exercises to enhance your emotional intelligence in combat.

CHAPTER SEVEN

The Holistic Approach of Lightsaber MMA

Understanding the Comprehensive Benefits
  - The Integration of Physical and Mental Fitness
  - Enhancing Emotional Well-being Through Training
  - Building a Supportive and Inclusive Community
  - Personal Growth and Self-Discovery

Subsection: Understanding the Comprehensive Benefits

1. *The Integration of Physical and Mental Fitness*

Lightsaber MMA is not just a physical discipline; it's a holistic journey that integrates mental fitness with physical prowess. This integration is key to the holistic approach of Lightsaber MMA, providing a balanced and comprehensive training experience.

"The Fusion of Body and Mind: Lightsaber MMA's Unique Approach"

Lightsaber MMA is a discipline that uniquely combines physical exercises with mental challenges, creating a holistic approach to personal development.

The Symbiosis of Physical and Mental Training:

Lightsaber MMA is not just about physical prowess; it's a blend of body and mind. Picture a duelist in training, engaging in rigorous physical drills, each movement precise and deliberate. These exercises are more than just a test of strength or agility; they are designed to challenge the mind, to develop a heightened sense of awareness and concentration.

Mental Challenges in Combat:

Amid a duel, a Lightsaber MMA practitioner is not only battling an opponent but also their mental tiers. Quick decision-making, strategic planning and adaptability are as crucial as physical skills. Each encounter is a mental puzzle, requiring the duelist to read the opponent's intentions, anticipate movements, and react not just with their body but with their mind.

Meditation and Mindfulness:

Integral to Lightsaber MMA is the practice of meditation and mindfulness. These techniques, often incorporated at the beginning or end of a training session, enhance focus, reduce stress, and improve emotional regulation. This mental discipline is essential for duelists, enabling them to enter a state of calm alertness, crucial during high-stakes competitions.

The Role of Visualization:

Visualization is another powerful tool in Lightsaber MMA. Practitioners are encouraged to mentally rehearse their movements, strategies, and combats. This mental practice strengthens neural pathways, enhancing muscle memory and preparing the mind for actual physical engagement. It's a process that hones not just the body but the mind's ability to strategize and execute.

Stress Management and Resilience:

Lightsaber MMA puts its practitioners in high-pressure scenarios. Managing this stress is as important as mastering physical skills. This discipline teaches how to remain composed under pressure, to channel stress into focus, and to turn challenges into opportunities for growth. This resilience is invaluable, both in and out of the arena.

Emotional Intelligence in Combat:

Understanding and managing emotions are key components of Lightsaber MMA. Practitioners learn to read their emotions during combat, transforming potential weaknesses such as fear or anger into strengths. This emotional intelligence is crucial for maintaining control and making clear-headed decisions during intense duels.

Cognitive Flexibility and Adaptation:

The unpredictable nature of Lightsaber MMA combats demands cognitive flexibility. Practitioners must be able to adapt quickly, changing tactics as the situation evolves. This flexibility is a mental skill, developed through the constant challenge of new and diverse training scenarios.

Community Learning and Mental Growth:

Finally, the Lightsaber MMA community plays a significant role in mental development. Practitioners learn from each other, sharing strategies, experiences, and insights. This collaborative environment fosters a growth mindset, encouraging continuous learning and mental expansion.

Lightsaber MMA is a discipline that transcends the physical realm, deeply engaging the mind. It's a journey that challenges practitioners to harmonize their physical skills with mental acuity, leading to comprehensive growth. As you embark on this path, embrace the mental challenges as much as the physical ones, for it is in the fusion of body and mind that true mastery lies.

"Transformative Journeys: The Life-Altering Impact of Lightsaber MMA"

This unique discipline isn't just about wielding a lightsaber; it's a path to personal transformation.

Confidence and Self-Esteem:
Consider the story of a young professional, once shy and unsure, who took up Lightsaber MMA. The discipline demanded not only physical strength but also mental resilience. Over time, the clarity and focus required in training began to seep into other aspects of their life. At work, their newfound confidence led to taking on more challenging projects, and in personal life, it meant healthier relationships and a stronger sense of self-worth.

Physical Health and Fitness:
Another individual, struggling with weight issues and a sedentary lifestyle, found a passion for fitness through Lightsaber MMA. The training sessions, demanding yet exhilarating, transformed their attitude towards physical health. They lost weight, gained muscle tone, and most importantly, developed a sustainable lifestyle that prioritizes health and well-being.

Stress Management:

In the high-pressure world we live in, Lightsaber MMA has become a sanctuary for many. One such story is of a corporate executive battling with stress and burnout. The rhythmic, focused nature of lightsaber drills, combined with the physical exertion, became a powerful tool for stress relief. They found in Lightsaber MMA a practice that not only challenges the body but also calms the mind.

Improved Focus and Concentration:

A university student, struggling with attention and focus, turned to Lightsaber MMA. The discipline required to master the forms and techniques significantly improved their concentration levels. This newfound focus was reflected in their academic performance, leading to better grades and a more enriching educational experience.

Community and Social Interaction:

Lightsaber MMA isn't just an individual journey. It's about being part of a community. Take the example of someone who moved to a new city and felt isolated. Joining a Lightsaber MMA club provided them with a sense of belonging. The friendships and connections formed in the training sessions extended beyond the studio, creating a supportive and engaging social network.

Enhanced Problem-Solving Skills:

Strategic thinking is a key element in Lightsaber MMA. One practitioner, a software developer, found that the strategic and tactical thinking in lightsaber combat translated into improved problem-solving skills at work. Analyzing combat scenarios helped sharpen their ability to navigate complex coding challenges.

Emotional Balance and Resilience:

For those battling emotional turmoil, Lightsaber MMA has been a path to stability and strength. An individual dealing with anxiety found that the discipline required in training helped in managing their emotional responses. The physical exertion provided an outlet for pent-up emotions, while the mindfulness aspect of the training helped in developing a more balanced emotional state.

Lightsaber MMA is a transformative experience. It empowers individuals with confidence, physical fitness, stress relief, focus, community bonds, strategic thinking, and emotional resilience. Each person's journey is unique, but the common thread is the profound positive impact Lightsaber MMA has on their lives.

"Mental Fitness: The Secret Weapon in Lightsaber Combat Mastery"

I want to talk about the vital role of mental fitness in enhancing physical performance in lightsaber combat. Just as the lightsaber is an extension of the body, mental fitness is an extension of physical prowess in this unique martial art.

Mind-Body Connection:

In lightsaber combat, the synergy between mind and body is paramount. The combatant must possess not only physical agility but also mental acuity. Picture this: During a duel, it's the mental clarity and focus that allow you to anticipate your opponent's next move, leading to a swift and effective response. The synchronization of mind and body is what turns a good combatant into a great one.

Emotional Regulation:

The art of lightsaber combat demands a high level of emotional control. It's not just about reacting to the opponent but doing so with a calm and composed mind. I've seen individuals who have harnessed this ability to remain tranquil under pressure, translating to more thoughtful and precise maneuvers in combat. Their ability to regulate emotions directly correlates with improved performance.

Visualization Techniques:

Mental rehearsal is a powerful tool in lightsaber combat. By visualizing sequences and outcomes, combatants prime their minds and bodies for success. This method of mental training sharpens reaction times and enhances strategic planning. Imagine a combatant who, before stepping onto the field, closes their eyes and visualizes each step, each swing, each parry – they're not just practicing, they're programming their mind for victory.

The Role of Concentration:

In lightsaber combat, a momentary lapse in concentration can be the difference between triumph and defeat. The ability to focus intensely and block out distractions is a product of mental fitness. Practitioners who train their minds to focus can better handle the intense concentration lightsaber combat demands, leading to enhanced performance.

Resilience and Grit:

Mental toughness is key in overcoming setbacks in training and combat. The journey of a lightsaber combatant is filled with challenges, and it's their mental resilience that helps them persevere. Those who develop this grit find that it not only helps them push through difficult training sessions but also faces their opponents with unwavering determination.

The Power of Mindfulness:

Mindfulness practices, such as meditation and breathing exercises, are incredibly beneficial. They aid in creating a heightened sense of awareness – both of self and the environment. This awareness is crucial in lightsaber combat, where being attuned to subtle shifts in your opponent's stance or the slightest change in their grip can give you the upper hand.

Continuous Learning and Adaptability:

Finally, mental fitness fosters a mindset of continuous learning and adaptability. The best lightsaber combatants are those who keep their minds open to new strategies and techniques, constantly adapting and evolving. They understand that mental flexibility is as important as physical agility.

While physical training forms the foundation of lightsaber combat, it's the mental fitness that truly elevates a combatant's skill. By focusing on developing mental clarity, emotional regulation, concentration, resilience, mindfulness, and adaptability, practitioners of Lightsaber MMA can achieve a level of mastery that transcends physical boundaries. In the arena of lightsaber combat, your mind is your most powerful weapon. Train it well, and you will find yourself not just performing but excelling in ways you never thought possible.

"Integrating Cognitive Challenges into Lightsaber MMA Training: A Guide to Enhanced Performance"

Let's dive into how we can enhance Lightsaber MMA training by integrating cognitive challenges into physical routines. This combination not only sharpens the body but also the mind, creating a holistic approach to training.

Scenario-Based Drills:

Imagine practicing lightsaber combat where each session is based on different scenarios. These drills require quick decision-making, and adapting strategies to changing circumstances. For example, participants might have to defend against multiple opponents or adjust to environmental constraints. This encourages strategic thinking and adaptability, critical skills in both Lightsaber MMA and life.

Memory and Pattern Recognition Exercises:

Incorporate exercises that challenge memory and pattern recognition. This could be as simple as memorizing complex lightsaber sequences or recognizing and responding to specific attack patterns from opponents. These exercises enhance concentration and mental agility, crucial for mastering lightsaber combat.

Reaction Time Training:

Incorporate exercises that unexpectedly change rhythms or patterns, requiring combatants to adjust quickly. This could involve switching from offensive to defensive tactics without notice or responding to visual or audio cues. Improving reaction time is essential for real-time strategy adjustments in Lightsaber MMA.

Mental Endurance Challenges:

Just as we train our bodies for physical endurance, we must train our minds for mental endurance. Extend training sessions or introduce elements of fatigue to test mental resilience. This simulates the pressures of an actual combat situation, where maintaining focus and strategy under stress is key.

Mindfulness and Focus Techniques:

Integrate mindfulness practices into the training regimen. Start or end sessions with meditation to enhance focus and mental clarity. Practicing mindfulness can significantly improve concentration, allowing combatants to remain present and composed during intense lightsaber battles.

Tactical Problem-Solving Activities:

Engage in activities that require tactical problem-solving. Set up combat scenarios where participants must find creative ways to overcome disadvantages such as limited mobility or outnumbered situations. This fosters innovative thinking and strategic planning, vital for Lightsaber MMA.

Team-Based Strategic Exercises:

Incorporate team-based drills that require collective strategizing and execution. This not only improves individual cognitive skills but also enhances communication and teamwork. In Lightsaber MMA, understanding how to work effectively with others can be a game-changer.

Post-Training Reflection and Analysis:

Finally, encourage post-training reflection and analysis. Discussing what went well, what didn't, and why, helps in understanding the thought processes behind actions. This reflective practice not only solidifies learning but also encourages continuous improvement and strategic refinement.

By integrating cognitive challenges into Lightsaber MMA physical training routines, we create a more comprehensive training experience. This approach not only prepares combatants physically but also mentally, equipping them with the skills necessary for both the arena and life. Remember, in Lightsaber MMA, the mind is as powerful a tool as the body. Train it well, and you'll see remarkable improvements in your performance. Keep pushing your limits, and remember – the only limit is the one you set yourself.

2. Enhancing Emotional Well-being Through Training

Training in Lightsaber MMA also offers significant benefits for emotional well-being. It's a discipline that encourages self-expression, stress relief, and emotional resilience.

"Harnessing Lightsaber MMA Training as a Healthy Outlet for Stress and Emotional Expression"

In today's fast-paced world, where stress is a constant companion, finding a physical activity that not only challenges the body but also calms the mind is critical. Lightsaber MMA training offers just that—a dynamic, engaging, and profoundly therapeutic experience.

Physical Release of Stress:
At the core of Lightsaber MMA training is the physical exertion it demands. Engaging in intense physical activity is a proven stress reliever. As you learn to wield the lightsaber, focusing on technique and form, your mind gets a break from daily worries. The physical effort releases endorphins, the body's natural mood lifters, leading to a state of euphoria often referred to as the 'runner's high'. This biochemical shift reduces stress and enhances overall well-being.

Mindfulness and Present Moment Awareness:
Lightsaber MMA requires a high level of present-moment awareness. As you focus on your movements and your opponent's actions, you enter a state of mindfulness. This presence stops the constant stream of thoughts,

especially those related to past worries or future anxieties, offering mental relief and clarity.

Emotional Expression and Release:

In Lightsaber MMA, each strike and defensive move is an opportunity to express and release pent-up emotions. The controlled environment allows for the safe expression of aggression, frustration, and even anger. Channeling these emotions through the discipline of martial arts provides a healthy way to cope with negative feelings, transforming them into positive actions.

The Discipline of Routine and Structure:

Regular training provides structure, which is therapeutic for those feeling overwhelmed by life's unpredictability. The discipline required to master Lightsaber MMA techniques offers a sense of control and achievement. Consistent practice instills a routine that can bring stability and predictability, which are calming during tumultuous times.

Community Support and Social Interaction:

Lightsaber MMA training is not just about individual skills; it's also about being part of a community. The camaraderie experienced during training sessions fosters social support, an essential element in stress reduction. Sharing experiences, challenges, and successes with fellow practitioners creates a sense of belonging and mutual understanding, reducing feelings of isolation.

Confidence and Self-Empowerment:

As practitioners progress in their training, they experience a boost in self-confidence and empowerment. Overcoming physical and mental challenges in training reinforces a sense of accomplishment. This empowerment spills over into other areas of life, providing a solid foundation to tackle stress with a positive mindset.

Enhancing Focus and Concentration:
The complex techniques and strategies of Lightsaber MMA demand intense focus and concentration. This requirement to concentrate on a single task is a form of mental training that enhances overall cognitive abilities, including attention and focus. A focused mind is better equipped to handle stress, as it can more effectively process and react to challenging situations.

Lightsaber MMA training is a holistic approach to wellness. It provides a unique blend of physical exertion, mental focus, emotional release, and community support, making it an ideal practice for those seeking a healthy outlet for stress and emotional expression. The journey to self-improvement is ongoing, and integrating practices like Lightsaber MMA into your life can be a powerful tool in managing stress and fostering emotional well-being. Stay focused, stay driven, and let your training be your sanctuary.

"Transforming Lives: Emotional Well-being Through Lightsaber MMA"

Let's delve into the transformative stories of individuals who've found a path to improved emotional well-being through the discipline and practice of Lightsaber MMA.

The Journey of Self-Discovery
One practitioner's journey began in the throes of depression. Struggling with self-esteem and feeling disconnected, they

stumbled upon a Lightsaber MMA class. Initially skeptical, they soon found themselves immersed in the rhythmic movements and the community's warmth. The physical exercise became a conduit for releasing pent-up emotions, while the discipline required for mastering techniques provided a sense of accomplishment and progress. Over time, they noticed a significant shift in their mood and outlook. The focus required in lightsaber MMA helped them gain clarity and understand their emotional triggers better, leading to a newfound sense of self-awareness and confidence.

Overcoming Anxiety with Graceful Combat

Another individual was grappling with anxiety and panic attacks. Seeking a non-traditional method of coping, they took up Lightsaber MMA. The precise, controlled movements required in the practice demanded full concentration, which gradually helped in easing their anxious thoughts. The supportive environment of the dojo provided a safe space to express and manage their anxiety. The mastery of each new skill in lightsaber MMA boosted their self-esteem, and the physical exertion was instrumental in mitigating anxiety symptoms. They found that the physical and mental discipline of lightsaber combat translated into an increased ability to manage stress and anxiety in daily life.

Building Resilience Through Martial Arts

A third story comes from someone who experienced significant loss and grief. Searching for a way to channel their emotions, they found solace in Lightsaber MMA. The practice became a physical expression of their inner turmoil. With every strike and parry, they were able to externalize the grief that felt so overwhelming internally. The community aspect of the training also played a critical role, offering a sense of belonging and understanding. Through regular training, they built resilience, learning to channel emotions into focused actions. The intense focus required in Lightsaber MMA helped them stay grounded and present, providing a break from the cycle of grief and despair.

From Isolation to Inclusion

The final story is about someone who felt isolated due to social anxiety. The inclusive nature of the Lightsaber MMA community was a revelation. Training alongside others with similar interests created a sense of belonging that had been missing in their life. Gradually, as they interacted more within the community and gained proficiency in the martial art, their social anxiety diminished. The dojo became a haven where they could be themselves without fear of judgment. The sense of achievement in mastering complex techniques helped in building their confidence, not just in the dojo, but in social situations outside of it.

These stories demonstrate the profound impact that Lightsaber MMA can have on emotional well-being. It's not just about physical fitness; it's a journey of mental and emotional fortification. As a coach and motivator, I believe in the power of physical disciplines like Lightsaber MMA to transform lives, offering a pathway to self-discovery, resilience, and emotional healing. Every journey starts with a single step, and sometimes, that step is picking up a lightsaber and facing your inner battles.

"Emotional Intelligence and Resilience: The Lightsaber MMA Journey"

Lightsaber MMA and its incredible role in developing emotional intelligence and resilience.

Emotional Intelligence in the Dojo

Lightsaber MMA is not just about physical agility; it's a profound journey into self-awareness and emotional mastery. The dojo becomes a microcosm of life's challenges, where practitioners learn to understand and regulate their emotions. Through the intricate dance of attack and defense, individuals confront not just their opponents but their inner fears, frustrations, and anxieties. This martial art teaches them to remain calm under pressure and to think clearly amidst chaos. Practitioners learn to read their opponents' emotions and intentions, developing empathy and social skills crucial both inside and outside the dojo.

Resilience through Rigorous Training

In Lightsaber MMA, resilience is forged in the fires of rigorous training. Each session is a test of endurance, pushing individuals to their limits and beyond. The journey is filled with setbacks – missed strikes, lost matches, and physical exhaustion. Yet, it's these very challenges that build resilience. Practitioners learn the art of bouncing back, turning failures into stepping stones for success. The path to mastery in Lightsaber MMA is a lesson in perseverance, teaching the invaluable life skill of enduring and overcoming adversity.

Mindfulness and Emotional Control

One of the most profound lessons in Lightsaber MMA is mindfulness. Amidst the whirl of combat, practitioners learn to center themselves, to be fully present in the moment. This heightened state of awareness extends beyond physical movements to emotional control. Practitioners learn to recognize their emotional responses – the surge of adrenaline, the flutter of anxiety – and to manage them effectively. This emotional control is a powerful tool, enhancing decision-making skills and fostering a balanced mind.

Empathy and Connection

Lightsaber MMA also cultivates empathy. By training with diverse partners, individuals learn to understand and respect different perspectives and emotions. This martial art fosters a deep sense of connection and community, where practitioners support and uplift each other. The dojo becomes a space of shared experiences and mutual growth, where emotional intelligence flourishes.

Stress Relief and Emotional Expression

The practice of Lightsaber MMA is a dynamic outlet for stress. The physical exertion is cathartic, allowing for the release of pent-up emotions. The discipline of the sport provides a structured way to express and manage emotions, channeling energy into focused and constructive action. Practitioners often find that Lightsaber MMA becomes a sanctuary, a place where they can shed the weight of their daily stresses and emerge rejuvenated.

Lightsaber MMA equips individuals with emotional intelligence and resilience – skills that are vital in navigating the complexities of life. The dojo is not just a training ground for martial arts; it's a classroom for life, where each lesson in emotional control, resilience, empathy, and stress management prepares individuals for the challenges beyond its walls. Embrace this journey, and discover the transformative power of emotional intelligence and resilience in Lightsaber MMA. Every strike, every parry, is a step towards a stronger, more resilient you.

3. *Building a Supportive and Inclusive Community*

The holistic approach of Lightsaber MMA extends to fostering a supportive and inclusive community. This community is a crucial component of the discipline, providing a space for shared learning, encouragement, and camaraderie.

"The Power of Community in Lightsaber MMA"

The critical role of community in the holistic world of Lightsaber MMA.

Fostering a Sense of Belonging

The first and foremost element in Lightsaber MMA is the sense of community. This isn't just a group of individuals practicing a sport; it's a family. The dojo becomes a place where people of all backgrounds unite with a common passion. It's a melting pot of cultures, ideas, and experiences, fostering a strong sense of belonging and identity. Within this community, everyone is valued, everyone's voice matters, and this inclusiveness is paramount for personal and collective growth.

Collective Growth and Learning

In the realm of Lightsaber MMA, each practitioner's growth is intertwined with that of others. The community offers a diverse range of perspectives and skills, enabling members to learn from one another. Beginners and veterans alike share the floor, exchanging techniques and insights. This collaborative learning environment accelerates skill development and fosters a culture of continuous improvement.

Support and Encouragement

One of the most beautiful aspects of the Lightsaber MMA community is the unwavering support and encouragement it offers. The path of martial arts is fraught with challenges and setbacks. It's in these moments that the community becomes a pillar of strength. There's always someone to lift you when you fall, to cheer you on when you succeed, and to push you beyond your perceived limits. This supportive network is instrumental in building resilience and confidence.

Emotional and Mental Well-being

The community aspect of Lightsaber MMA extends beyond physical training. It becomes a haven for emotional and mental well-being. Practitioners often find solace in their peers, sharing not just their triumphs but also their struggles. The dojo becomes a space of empathy, understanding, and healing, where individuals can express themselves freely and find comfort in camaraderie.

A Platform for Leadership and Contribution

Lightsaber MMA communities are also breeding grounds for leadership. They offer countless opportunities for individuals to step up and contribute. Whether it's leading a class, organizing events, or mentoring newcomers, these roles foster a sense of responsibility and pride. Practitioners learn to lead with integrity and compassion, skills that transcend the dojo and apply to all areas of life.

Cultural Exchange and Diversity

The diversity within Lightsaber MMA communities is a goldmine for cultural exchange and understanding. People from different walks of life come together, sharing their unique traditions and experiences. This cultural richness adds depth to the practice, making it a truly global and inclusive art form.

A Community of Warriors

The community within Lightsaber MMA is not just an add-on; it's the heart and soul of the practice. It's a sanctuary where individuals grow not just as martial artists but as human beings. The lessons learned in this community – of empathy, support, resilience, and leadership – resonate far beyond the dojo. They shape practitioners into well-rounded, compassionate individuals ready to face the world. So, embrace your community, contribute to it, and watch as it transforms not just your practice, but your life.

In the journey of Lightsaber MMA, you're never alone. You're part of a community – a family of warriors – and that's your greatest strength.

"The Supportive Force of the Lightsaber MMA Community"

Remarkable ways in which the Lightsaber MMA community supports and uplifts its members, creating an environment of growth and positivity.

Empowering Each Other Through Challenges

In Lightsaber MMA, every challenge faced is an opportunity for the community to come together. When a member struggles with a particular technique or faces a personal hurdle, the community steps in. It's not just about providing tips or technical advice, but also about offering emotional support and encouragement. This collective approach to problem-solving not only helps overcome the immediate challenge but also strengthens the bonds within the community.

Celebrating Successes Together

Every victory, no matter how small is a cause for celebration in the Lightsaber MMA community. Whether it's mastering a new move, winning a sparring match, or achieving a personal fitness goal, these moments are shared and celebrated by all. This culture of acknowledgment and appreciation boosts confidence and motivates members to set and achieve higher goals.

Mentorship and Guidance

Experienced practitioners often take on mentorship roles, offering guidance and insights to newcomers. This mentor-mentee relationship is pivotal in Lightsaber MMA, as it fosters a sense of belonging and accelerates learning. The mentors provide not just technical training but also life lessons, helping mentees navigate both the world of Lightsaber MMA and personal challenges.

A Safe Space for Expression and Growth

The Lightsaber MMA community is a haven where members can express themselves without fear of judgment. It's a space where they can explore their capabilities, push their limits, and discover new aspects of their personalities. This freedom of expression is crucial for personal growth, self-discovery, and building self-esteem.

Fostering Resilience Through Peer Support

Life can be tough, and sometimes, the battles we face are outside the dojo. The Lightsaber MMA community understands this and stands as a solid support system for its members. Whether it's dealing with a loss, facing a professional setback, or battling personal demons, the community provides a supportive ear, a shoulder to lean on, and words of wisdom, fostering resilience and helping members bounce back stronger.

Diversity and Inclusion

One of the most beautiful aspects of the Lightsaber MMA community is its diversity and inclusiveness. It welcomes people from all walks of life, irrespective of their background, age, or skill level. This diversity enriches the community, as members learn to respect and appreciate different perspectives and cultures, which in turn fosters a sense of global unity and understanding.

Social Events and Gatherings

The community often organizes social events and gatherings outside the dojo. These events are crucial for building camaraderie, strengthening friendships, and creating lasting memories. They serve as a reminder that the community is not just about training and combat; it's about forming meaningful connections and having fun together.

A Community of Strength and Support.

The Lightsaber MMA community is more than a group of martial arts enthusiasts; it's a family. It's a place where individuals come together to share, learn, and grow, both as martial artists and as human beings. The support, mentorship, and camaraderie found in this community are unparalleled, making it a powerful force in the lives of its members. In Lightsaber MMA, you're never alone; you're part of a community that supports you, uplifts you, and celebrates you. So, cherish this community, contribute to it, and let it be your strength as you journey through the world of Lightsaber MMA and beyond.

"The Power of Diversity and Inclusion in Martial Arts Communities"

The profound benefits of being part of a diverse and inclusive martial arts community are a topic close to my heart. Martial arts, in its essence, are not just about physical prowess; it's a journey of personal growth, and being part of a diverse community significantly enriches this journey.

Enriched Learning Experience

In a diverse martial arts community, you're exposed to a variety of styles, techniques, and philosophies. This eclectic mix is not just intellectually stimulating; it provides a comprehensive learning experience. You're not just learning how to execute a move; you're understanding its origin, its cultural significance, and its variations. This depth of learning fosters a deeper appreciation and respect for martial arts as a whole.

Breaking Down Cultural Barriers

Martial arts have always been a bridge between cultures. In a diverse community, you interact with people from different backgrounds, each bringing their unique perspectives and experiences. These interactions are instrumental in breaking down cultural stereotypes and prejudices, fostering a sense of global unity and mutual respect.

Enhanced Creativity and Innovation

Diversity breeds creativity. When you train with people of different backgrounds, you're exposed to various ways of thinking and problem-solving. This exposure can significantly enhance your creativity, both in and out of the dojo. You're more likely to think outside the box, approach challenges differently, and innovate.

Personal Growth and Empathy

Training in a diverse environment fosters empathy and emotional intelligence. You become more aware of the challenges others face, understand different viewpoints, and learn to communicate effectively with a broad range of people. This growth in emotional intelligence is invaluable, not just in martial arts but in every aspect of life.

A Stronger Sense of Community

A diverse and inclusive community is a strong community. When people from different walks of life come together with a common goal, they form deep bonds. These bonds are fortified by mutual respect, shared experiences, and collective growth. In such a community, you're not just a practitioner; you're part of a family that supports, encourages, and uplifts each other.

Better Conflict Resolution Skills

Martial arts is fundamentally about discipline and control, including conflict resolution. In a diverse community, you're more likely to encounter differing opinions and perspectives. Learning to navigate these differences amicably and respectfully is a valuable skill that martial arts training in a diverse setting can enhance.

Preparing for Global Challenges

We live in a globalized world, and the ability to interact effectively with people from various backgrounds is essential. Training in a diverse martial arts community prepares you for this reality. It equips you with the skills to communicate, collaborate, and lead in an increasingly interconnected world.

A Microcosm of the World

Being part of a diverse and inclusive martial arts community is incredibly beneficial. It's a microcosm of the world – a place where different cultures, ideas, and perspectives come together to create something beautiful and powerful. In this community, you're not just honing your physical skills; you're cultivating a deeper understanding of humanity, fostering respect for diversity, and developing into a well-rounded individual.

4. Personal Growth and Self-Discovery

A key aspect of the holistic approach of Lightsaber MMA is its focus on personal growth and self-discovery. Practitioners are encouraged to explore their limits, discover new strengths, and learn more about themselves through training.

"Igniting Personal Growth and Self-Discovery Through Lightsaber MMA Training"

A fascinating journey of self-improvement and discovery: Lightsaber MMA training. This unique blend of martial arts isn't just about physical fitness; it's a gateway to personal growth and self-discovery.

Cultivating Discipline and Focus

Lightsaber MMA training requires a high level of discipline. This discipline transcends the dojo and seeps into every aspect of life. It teaches you to focus on your goals, manage your time effectively, and develop a strong work ethic. It's not just about mastering the lightsaber; it's about mastering your life.

Building Confidence and Self-Esteem

Engaging in Lightsaber MMA training empowers you. As you learn new techniques and witness your skills improving, your confidence soars. This increased self-esteem is pivotal. It enables you to take on challenges with a belief in your abilities, not just in training, but in all areas of life.

Learning the Art of Resilience

In Lightsaber MMA, you face challenges and setbacks. Each time you're knocked down, you learn to get back up. This resilience is invaluable. Life will throw punches, and the ability to bounce back stronger is a testament to the power of this training.

Enhancing Self-awareness

Through Lightsaber MMA, you become more in tune with your body and mind. You learn to understand your strengths and weaknesses, both physically and mentally. This self-awareness is the first step in personal growth. Knowing who you are is essential to knowing who you want to become.

Developing Emotional Intelligence

In the heat of combat, controlling your emotions is crucial. Lightsaber MMA training teaches you to manage stress, anger, and fear. This emotional intelligence is critical for personal and professional relationships. You learn to respond, not react, making you a better communicator and leader.

Fostering Social Connections

Lightsaber MMA is not a solitary journey. You train with others, learn from them, and grow together. These social connections are a bedrock for personal development. You learn empathy, cooperation, and the value of diverse perspectives.

Encouraging Continuous Learning

This journey is never-ending. There's always a new technique to master, a new challenge to overcome. This mindset of continuous learning is pivotal for personal growth. It keeps you humble, curious and always striving for improvement.

Aligning Body, Mind, and Spirit

Finally, Lightsaber MMA aligns your physical, mental, and spiritual aspects. It's a holistic approach to personal development. As your body grows stronger, your mind becomes sharper, and your spirit more resilient. This harmony is essential for a fulfilled, balanced life.

Transformation

Lightsaber MMA training is more than a physical discipline; it's a catalyst for personal transformation. It's a journey that challenges you, changes you, and ultimately leads you to a deeper understanding of yourself.

"Igniting Transformation: Personal Journeys of Self-Realization through Lightsaber MMA"

Incredible stories of transformation and self-realization that I've come across in the world of Lightsaber MMA. These are not just stories about physical prowess; they're about personal journeys that have reshaped lives.

Embracing New Challenges

There's a story of a young professional who felt stuck in the monotony of everyday life. Lightsaber MMA presented a new challenge, an unfamiliar territory that pushed boundaries. The training required not just physical strength but mental agility. It wasn't long before this individual realized that the biggest battles were fought within, leading to profound self-awareness and a renewed zest for life.

Overcoming Personal Obstacles

Another story is of someone who struggled with self-doubt and anxiety. Lightsaber MMA training became a sanctuary, a place to confront inner fears. Each duel was more than a physical encounter; it was a step towards overcoming personal barriers. This journey wasn't just about learning to wield a lightsaber; it was about wielding inner strength to conquer personal demons.

Building Resilience and Perseverance

Consider the tale of an individual recovering from a major setback in life. Lightsaber MMA offered a structured path to regain confidence. Each training session was a lesson in resilience, teaching how to get back up after being knocked down, both literally and metaphorically. This path led to an incredible transformation from vulnerability to unwavering strength.

Discovering Community and Belonging

Then, there's a story of someone who felt isolated and disconnected. The Lightsaber MMA community provided a sense of belonging and a supportive environment where everyone was united by a common passion. This camaraderie went beyond the dojo; it fostered deep connections and lifelong friendships, filling a void of loneliness with the warmth of companionship.

Achieving Physical and Mental Balance

Another inspiring story is of an individual who struggled with maintaining a healthy lifestyle. Lightsaber MMA training brought discipline, not just in physical routines but also in mental and emotional aspects. This holistic approach led to a balanced life, with improved health, clearer focus, and greater emotional stability.

Unleashing Inner Potential

Lastly, there's the journey of someone who doubted their potential. Through Lightsaber MMA, they discovered strengths they never knew they had. The training pushed them beyond their perceived limits, leading to the realization that the only limits that exist are the ones we set for ourselves.

Profound Change

These stories are testaments to the transformative power of Lightsaber MMA. It's not just a sport; it's a journey of self-discovery and growth. It teaches discipline, resilience, and the importance of community. Most importantly, it shows us that we are capable of so much more than we ever thought possible.

"Empowering Lives Through Lightsaber MMA: A Journey to Confidence, Self-Awareness, and Life Skills"

I want to talk about the remarkable impact of Lightsaber MMA on personal confidence, self-awareness, and life skills. This isn't just a sport; it's a transformative experience that shapes lives.

Building Unshakeable Confidence

Let's start with confidence. Engaging in Lightsaber MMA isn't just about physical training; it's about stepping into a realm of courage and self-belief. Imagine someone who's always been hesitant, always doubting their abilities. Through the discipline of Lightsaber MMA, they find themselves in situations that challenge their limits. Every successful block and every strategic move builds a layer of confidence. It's about realizing, "I can do this. I am capable." This newfound confidence transcends the dojo; it permeates every aspect of life.

Cultivating Profound Self-Awareness

Then there's self-awareness. Lightsaber MMA is like a mirror reflecting one's inner self. It's not just about knowing how to strike or defend; it's about understanding one's reactions, emotions, and thoughts under pressure. Participants learn to observe their feelings without judgment, leading to profound self-awareness. It's about recognizing personal strengths and areas for growth, both in the arena and in life.

Mastering Crucial Life Skills

Lightsaber MMA is also an incredible teacher of life skills. Think about someone who's struggled with focus and discipline. The structured training and the need for strategic thinking in Lightsaber MMA provide a framework for developing these essential skills. There's also the aspect of resilience – getting knocked down and getting back up, both literally and metaphorically. This resilience becomes a critical life skill, helping individuals face personal and professional challenges with a steadfast spirit.

Enhancing Emotional Intelligence

Emotional intelligence is another key area where Lightsaber MMA makes a significant impact. Participants learn to control their emotions during high-stress duels, a skill that is invaluable in daily life. It's about managing anger, frustration, and even excitement – channeling these emotions in a way that's productive and not destructive.

Fostering Leadership and Teamwork

Lightsaber MMA also teaches leadership and teamwork. In group training and sparring sessions, participants learn to communicate, collaborate, and lead. These are skills that enhance their professional and personal relationships, promoting a sense of community and mutual respect.

Encouraging Continuous Personal Growth

Finally, Lightsaber MMA is a journey of continuous personal growth. It's not about being the best in the room; it's about being better than you were yesterday. This mindset of growth and improvement is invaluable. It encourages lifelong learning and adaptability, qualities that are essential in our ever-changing world.

A Holistic Approach to Personal Development

Lightsaber MMA is much more than a physical discipline; it's a holistic approach to personal development. It builds confidence, self-awareness, and essential life skills. It teaches emotional intelligence, leadership, and the value of teamwork. Most importantly, it instills a mindset of continuous growth and improvement. So, if you're on a journey of self-improvement, consider Lightsaber MMA not just as a sport, but as a pathway to a more empowered, aware, and skillful life.

CHAPTER EIGHT

Embarking on Your Lightsaber MMA Journey

Taking the First Steps
- Understanding the Basics of Lightsaber MMA
- Finding the Right Training Environment
- Setting Realistic Goals and Tracking Progress
- Engaging with the Lightsaber MMA Community

Subsection: Taking the First Steps

1. *Understanding the Basics of Lightsaber MMA*

Embarking on your Lightsaber MMA journey begins with a solid understanding of the basics. This foundational knowledge is crucial for building your skills and appreciating the discipline's depth.

"Unleashing Your Potential: The Fundamental Principles and Techniques of Lightsaber MMA"

Lightsaber MMA is a discipline that not only enhances physical prowess but also fosters personal growth and empowerment. This exciting blend of martial arts offers more than just physical training; it's a journey towards self-mastery.

Understanding the Core Principles

At the heart of Lightsaber MMA lies a set of core principles – discipline, respect, and mindfulness. Discipline is fundamental; it's about showing up, committing to the training, and pushing beyond your comfort zone. Respect is crucial, not just for others but for oneself, honoring the body and mind as tools of personal development. Mindfulness, the third pillar, involves being present at the moment, and fully engaged with every movement and decision.

Mastering the Techniques

The techniques of Lightsaber MMA are a blend of traditional martial arts and modern combat strategies, adapted to the unique properties of a lightsaber. The training begins with basic stances and movements, focusing on agility, balance, and coordination. As you progress, you learn advanced techniques like parries, strikes, and combinations, requiring not just physical skill but strategic thinking.

Developing Strategic Thinking

Lightsaber MMA is not just about physical combat; it's a mental game. It requires anticipating the opponent's moves, understanding their strategy, and adapting swiftly. This strategic thinking is a skill that extends beyond the dojo – it's applicable in everyday life, enhancing decision-making and problem-solving abilities.

Enhancing Physical Fitness

The physical training involved in Lightsaber MMA is intense and comprehensive. It improves cardiovascular health, builds muscle strength, enhances flexibility, and boosts endurance. The dynamic nature of the training ensures a full-body workout, promoting overall physical fitness.

Building Mental Resilience

Mental resilience is a significant benefit of Lightsaber MMA. It teaches you to handle stress, manage emotions, and stay calm under pressure. This resilience is essential not only in combat but in facing life's challenges. It's about developing a mindset that sees obstacles as opportunities for growth.

Fostering Community and Support

Lightsaber MMA is not a solitary journey. It's practiced within a community of fellow enthusiasts, providing a supportive environment for learning and growth. This community aspect fosters a sense of belonging, offering encouragement, motivation, and camaraderie.

Embracing Continuous Improvement

One of the most beautiful aspects of Lightsaber MMA is the ethos of continuous improvement. It's not about being perfect; it's about being better than you were yesterday. This mindset fosters a lifelong journey of learning and self-improvement.

A Path to Empowerment

Lightsaber MMA is more than a physical discipline; it's a path to empowerment. It combines the physical with the mental, and the strategic with the intuitive, offering a holistic approach to personal development. Whether you're looking to improve your physical fitness, sharpen your mind, or find a supportive community, Lightsaber MMA provides a dynamic and fulfilling path to achieve these goals.

"Igniting the Spark: Early Learning Experiences of Seasoned Lightsaber MMA Practitioners"

Inspiring early learning experiences of seasoned practitioners in Lightsaber Mixed Martial Arts (MMA). Their journeys, filled with discovery and transformation, serve as powerful examples of growth, discipline, and the enduring spirit of a student.

Discovering Passion Amidst Challenges

One practitioner, who is now an acclaimed instructor, recalls their initial encounter with Lightsaber MMA. Despite having no prior martial arts background, they were captivated by the blend of physicality and artistry. Early challenges included mastering basic stances and movements, often leading to frustration. However, their passion for the sport and a supportive training community kept them going, transforming initial struggles into stepping stones for mastery.

The Mentor Who Shaped a Path

Another practitioner shares the pivotal role a mentor played in their early training. This mentor, renowned for their skill and wisdom, didn't just teach techniques but also imparted lessons on mental resilience and emotional balance. The practitioner credits these early lessons with shaping their approach to Lightsaber MMA and life, teaching them the importance of patience, focus, and respect for the art.

Overcoming Self-Doubt

A story that stands out is of a practitioner who initially doubted their ability to excel in Lightsaber MMA. Plagued by self-doubt, they struggled with coordination and agility in the early days. It was through persistent practice, reflective learning, and encouragement from fellow students that they began to see progress, eventually leading to a boost in confidence and skill.

The First Breakthrough

A memorable tale comes from a practitioner who experienced their first breakthrough during a sparring session. Initially, they found it challenging to anticipate opponents' moves and to counter effectively. However, a particular sparring session, where they successfully implemented a strategy learned in training, marked a significant turning point. This experience was a confidence booster, reinforcing the importance of strategic thinking and adaptability in Lightsaber MMA.

Learning the Value of Discipline

An experienced practitioner reflects on the early days of rigorous training routines. The discipline required for Lightsaber MMA was initially overwhelming, from maintaining physical fitness to dedicating hours to practice. However, this discipline soon became a way of life, teaching them the value of hard work, consistency, and dedication, not only in martial arts but also in personal and professional arenas.

The First Tournament Experience

The excitement and nerves of participating in their first Lightsaber MMA tournament are a common memory among practitioners. The experience of competing, dealing with the pressure, and learning from both victories and defeats provided invaluable lessons. These early competitions instilled a sense of sportsmanship, the importance of continuous learning, and the joy of being part of a larger community.

These stories from seasoned Lightsaber MMA practitioners highlight that the journey is as important as the destination. Their early experiences, filled with challenges, learning, and growth, paved the way for their success and mastery of the art. These narratives inspire us to embrace our beginnings, persevere through difficulties, and continuously evolve, both in our chosen fields and in life.

"Mastering the Basics: The Key to Advancing in Lightsaber MMA"

Let's talk about the profound importance of mastering basic concepts in any skill, especially in an intricate discipline like Lightsaber Mixed Martial Arts (MMA). The journey to mastery is not just about learning advanced techniques but fundamentally understanding and perfecting the basics.

Foundations for Growth

In Lightsaber MMA, as in life, strong foundations are crucial. Starting with the basics—stances, grips, and simple movements—is not just about learning these elements in isolation. It's about understanding how these foundational skills interconnect and form the backbone of more complex techniques. The basics are not just the first steps but the core pillars that support your entire journey.

Building Confidence and Competence

When practitioners focus on mastering the basics, they build confidence. There's a deep sense of accomplishment in perfecting a stance or a basic strike. This confidence then becomes the bedrock for approaching more complex techniques with a positive mindset. It's not just about learning movements; it's about cultivating a mindset of growth and confidence.

The Value of Precision and Control

Basic techniques in Lightsaber MMA are designed to teach precision and control. Every movement in martial arts is intentional. By focusing on basics, practitioners learn to control their bodies, understand their limits, and how to extend beyond them safely. This control is vital when progressing to more complex techniques, where precision is not just about skill but also about safety.

Understanding the Art

The beauty of Lightsaber MMA lies not just in its physicality but also in its artistry. The basics are not just techniques; they are the language through which the art speaks. By deeply understanding basic movements and stances, practitioners learn the language of Lightsaber MMA. This understanding is crucial for appreciating the art and for developing one's unique style within it.

Preparing for Challenges

In training, as in life, challenges are inevitable. A solid grasp of basic skills prepares practitioners for these challenges. Whether it's adapting to an opponent's style in a duel or overcoming a plateau in skill development, the basics provide the tools needed to navigate these challenges effectively. They offer a reliable foundation to return to, reassess, and build upon.

Long-term Success and Mastery

The pursuit of mastery in Lightsaber MMA is a long-term commitment. Mastering the basics is akin to building a strong, resilient foundation for a house. As techniques become more advanced, the stability of this foundation becomes increasingly important. Those who rush to advanced techniques without solidifying their basics often find themselves struggling later, having missed the crucial lessons that only the basics can teach.

The basics are far from basic. They are the essential building blocks for any practitioner aspiring to excel in Lightsaber MMA. By focusing on these fundamentals, practitioners not only set themselves up for success in advanced techniques but also cultivate a deeper understanding and appreciation for the art.

Start with beginner classes or online tutorials to learn the fundamentals of Lightsaber MMA.

2. Finding the Right Training Environment

Your growth in lightsaber MMA is significantly influenced by your training environment. It's essential to find a dojo or training group that aligns with your goals and values.

"Choosing the Right Training Environment: A Guide to Aligning with Your Learning Style and Objectives"

How to choose a training environment that not only suits your learning style but also aligns perfectly with your objectives, especially in disciplines like Lightsaber MMA or any other skill you're passionate about?

Understanding Your Learning Style

First and foremost, understand your learning style. Are you a visual learner who thrives on demonstrations? Or do you prefer a hands-on approach, learning by doing? Recognizing your learning style is crucial in selecting a training environment that complements and enhances your natural way of absorbing information.

Goal Alignment

Your training environment should align with your goals. Are you training for personal growth, or physical fitness, or aiming to compete professionally? Different training centers or coaches specialize in various aspects of training. Choose one that aligns with your objectives and can guide you toward achieving them.

The Importance of Culture and Atmosphere

The culture of the training environment plays a significant role in your development. A supportive, positive atmosphere not only boosts learning but also motivates you to push your limits. Look for a community that matches your values and attitude towards learning and growth.

Accessibility and Convenience

Consider the practical aspects such as location and scheduling. A conveniently located training center with flexible schedules can make a big difference in maintaining consistency, which is key to mastering any skill.

Quality of Instruction

The quality of instruction is paramount. Research the credentials and experience of the instructors. Are they skilled in adapting their teaching methods to suit different learning styles? Experienced and versatile instructors can tailor their approach to enhance your learning experience.

Opportunities for Practical Application

Ensure that the training environment offers ample opportunities for practical application, such as sparring sessions in

Lightsaber MMA. Real-world application of skills is crucial for comprehensive learning and improvement.

Feedback and Personal Attention

Feedback is a powerful tool for improvement. A training environment that offers constructive, personalized feedback can significantly enhance your learning curve. Look for instructors who are not just teachers but also mentors who can provide individual attention.

Facilities and Equipment

The quality of facilities and equipment should not be overlooked. Well-maintained, safe, and up-to-date equipment contributes to an effective learning environment. It also reflects the training center's commitment to providing the best for its students.

Community and Peer Learning

A supportive community and peer learning opportunities can greatly enhance your training experience. Learning from and alongside peers not only fosters a sense of community but also provides diverse perspectives and insights that enrich your learning.

Trial Classes

Finally, try before you commit. Many training centers offer trial classes. Participate in a few sessions to get a feel of the training environment, teaching style, and whether it aligns with your preferences and goals.

Choosing the right training environment is a personal decision that should be made with careful consideration of various factors including learning style, objectives, culture, quality of instruction, and practical aspects.

"Finding Your Ideal Training Ground: Stories of Accelerated Progress in Lightsaber MMA"

Exploring the power of finding your ideal training setting in the world of Lightsaber MMA, through the experiences of individuals who have seen remarkable progress by aligning their training with their unique needs and goals.

Recognizing Personal Needs

One practitioner's story begins with understanding her specific needs. She was someone who thrived in a structured, disciplined environment. After trying out several gyms, she discovered a Lightsaber MMA academy that emphasized a regimented training schedule, which perfectly aligned with her disciplined approach to learning. This congruence between her learning style and the training environment led to a significant improvement in her technique and confidence.

The Power of a Supportive Community

Another individual's journey highlights the importance of a supportive community. He was struggling with self-confidence and motivation. Upon joining a local Lightsaber MMA club known for its friendly and encouraging community, he found himself more motivated than ever. The positive reinforcement and camaraderie he experienced accelerated his learning curve and transformed his approach to training.

Adapting to Learning Styles

An inspiring story comes from a visual learner who was initially struggling in a traditional training setup. He discovered a training center that utilized advanced visual aids and demonstrations, making complex maneuvers easier to understand and replicate. This alignment with his learning style allowed him to grasp techniques more quickly and efficiently.

Flexibility and Customization

A young woman shared how finding a training center that offered customizable training programs was a game-changer for her. With a busy schedule, she needed flexibility. The academy she joined provided personalized training schedules and one-on-one sessions, which allowed her to train effectively despite her time constraints, leading to rapid improvements in her skills.

Emphasis on Mental Training

One practitioner's breakthrough came when he joined a Lightsaber MMA academy that placed equal emphasis on mental training. The holistic approach, focusing not just on physical skills but also on mental resilience and strategic thinking, played a crucial role in his overall development as a Lightsaber MMA fighter.

Access to Diverse Techniques

A man's journey illustrates the benefit of exposure to a wide range of fighting styles. He initially trained in a gym with a very narrow focus. Switching to a more diverse academy exposed him to various styles and techniques, broadening his skill set and strategic understanding of Lightsaber MMA.

Inspirational Mentors

Finally, a story that stands out is of a practitioner who was inspired by his mentor. The mentor's approach to teaching, which combined technical prowess with life lessons, deeply resonated with him. This mentorship not only improved his Lightsaber MMA skills but also his personal growth and approach to life's challenges.

These stories underscore a crucial point: finding the right training environment is a deeply personal journey and plays a critical role in one's growth and success in Lightsaber MMA. It's not just about the physical space but about the culture, teaching style, community, and alignment with personal goals and learning styles. When these elements come together, the progress is not just in skills, but in confidence, motivation, and overall personal development.

"The Empowering Journey of Lightsaber MMA Training in a Supportive, Challenging, and Respectful Environment"

The enlightening journey of Lightsaber MMA training within a nurturing environment that is simultaneously supportive, challenging, and respectful.

1. Cultivating a Supportive Atmosphere:

In the realm of Lightsaber MMA, a supportive environment is paramount. Imagine stepping into a space where your unique journey is not only acknowledged but celebrated. This type of setting fosters an empowering atmosphere, where encouragement and positive reinforcement are the norm. Such an environment enables learners to take risks, push their boundaries, and explore their capabilities without the fear of judgment.

2. Embracing Challenges as Opportunities:

In a challenging training environment, every obstacle becomes a stepping stone toward personal growth. Lightsaber MMA, with its intricate techniques and strategies, demands physical and mental agility. When presented with challenges in a supportive context, practitioners are more likely to embrace these hurdles as opportunities for learning and improvement. This approach not only enhances skill but also instills resilience and adaptability.

3. Respect as a Cornerstone:

Respect in training is not just about etiquette; it's about recognizing and valuing each individual's journey. A respectful Lightsaber MMA environment nurtures mutual understanding and empathy among practitioners. It creates a safe space where learners feel valued and heard, which is crucial for personal and communal growth. Respect also extends to self-respect, encouraging practitioners to honor their limits and listen to their bodies.

4. Personal Growth and Self-Discovery:

The combination of support, challenge, and respect in Lightsaber MMA training paves the way for profound personal growth and self-discovery. Practitioners often find themselves on a journey that goes beyond physical training; it becomes a path to discovering inner strengths, confronting personal fears, and developing a deeper sense of self-awareness.

5. Building Lasting Relationships:

Training in such an environment fosters a sense of community and camaraderie. As practitioners work together, facing challenges, and supporting each other, strong bonds are formed. These relationships often extend beyond the training space, providing a network of support and friendship that can be invaluable in all areas of life.

6. Enhanced Learning Experience:

The synergy of a supportive, challenging, and respectful environment significantly enhances the learning experience. Practitioners are more open to feedback, more engaged in the process and more motivated to excel. This holistic approach to training ensures that learning is not just effective but also enjoyable and fulfilling.

7. Empowerment and Confidence:
Regular training in such an environment inevitably leads to increased empowerment and confidence. Practitioners develop not only physical strength and skill but also a strong sense of self-efficacy. They learn to trust their abilities, make decisions under pressure, and handle life's challenges with greater confidence.

The benefits of training Lightsaber MMA in an environment that balances support, challenges, and respect are immense. It creates a transformative experience that extends well beyond physical training, touching on every aspect of personal development. This journey is not just about mastering martial arts; it's about embarking on a path of self-empowerment and holistic growth.

Research local dojos or online communities, and visit them to find the right fit for your Lightsaber MMA journey.

3. Setting Realistic Goals and Tracking Progress

Goal setting is a powerful tool in your Lightsaber MMA journey. It helps maintain focus, motivation, and a sense of direction in your training.

"Setting Achievable Yet Challenging Goals in Lightsaber MMA: A Path to Mastery and Personal Growth"

How to set achievable yet challenging goals in the exhilarating world of Lightsaber MMA. This journey isn't just about becoming proficient in martial arts; it's about self-improvement, discipline, and realizing your true potential.

1. Start with Clarity:

The first step in setting goals in Lightsaber MMA is clarity. What do you want to achieve? Is it mastering a particular set of moves, improving your reflexes, or competing in tournaments? Clear, specific goals provide a roadmap for your journey. It's like igniting your lightsaber - knowing its purpose and direction.

2. Balance Challenge and Realism:

Goals should stretch your abilities while remaining attainable. If you're a beginner, aiming to compete at an advanced level within a month isn't just unrealistic; it's setting yourself up for disappointment. Instead, set a goal that challenges you but is within the realm of possibility, like mastering the basic defensive techniques in three months.

3. Break Down Goals into Smaller Steps:

Achieving mastery in Lightsaber MMA is a journey made up of many small steps. Break down your larger goals into smaller, manageable tasks. For instance, if your goal is to improve your footwork, start by dedicating sessions to specific footwork drills. Celebrate these small victories – they are the building blocks of your success.

4. Incorporate Timelines and Benchmarks:

Setting timelines helps maintain momentum and focus. Establish realistic time frames for your goals and monitor your progress. Regularly assess your performance against these benchmarks. Are you on track? Do adjustments need to be made? This ongoing evaluation keeps your goals aligned with your growth.

5. Embrace a Growth Mindset:

In Lightsaber MMA, like in life, adopting a growth mindset is crucial. View challenges as opportunities for growth. If a particular technique is difficult, see it as a chance to develop resilience and patience. Embrace feedback, both from yourself and others, as a tool for improvement.

6. Accountability and Support:

Share your goals with your trainer or fellow practitioners. They can offer support, guidance, and accountability. Sometimes, the path to achieving a goal can be as simple as committing to regular practice sessions with a training partner.

7. Visualize Success:

Visualization is a powerful tool. Imagine yourself achieving your goals – feel the grip of your lightsaber as you execute a perfect move, hear the sound of applause at a competition, or feel the satisfaction of mastering a challenging technique. Visualization not only motivates but also prepares your mind and body for the real experience.

8. Adjust Goals as You Grow:

Goals are not set in stone. As you progress in your Lightsaber MMA journey, your needs and aspirations will evolve. Regularly reassess and adjust your goals to reflect your current level and future aspirations. Flexibility in goal-setting is key to continuous growth and motivation.

Setting achievable yet challenging goals in Lightsaber MMA is a dynamic and rewarding process. It requires clarity, realism, a step-by-step approach, timelines, a growth mindset, support, visualization, and adaptability.

"Harnessing the Power of Consistent Progress Tracking in Lightsaber MMA"

Let's dive into a crucial aspect of achieving success in any field, especially in the dynamic world of Lightsaber Mixed Martial Arts (MMA): consistent progress tracking.

Imagine you're embarking on a journey in Lightsaber MMA. It's a path that not only tests your physical abilities but also challenges your mental fortitude. In this journey, the role of consistent progress tracking cannot be overstated. It's like having a compass in the wilderness; it guides you, shows you how far you've come, and what more needs to be conquered.

Let's start by understanding the importance of setting clear, measurable goals in Lightsaber MMA. Whether it's mastering a new combat technique, increasing your stamina, or preparing for a tournament, each goal needs a roadmap. This is where progress tracking comes in. It allows you to break down these large goals into smaller, manageable milestones. Remember, success is the sum of small efforts, repeated day in and day out.

Now, consider the role of regular self-assessment in your training. This could be weekly reflections on your training sessions, noting improvements in your techniques, or areas needing more work. It's about being honest with yourself, recognizing your strengths, and being aware of your weaknesses. Self-assessment acts as a reality check and keeps you grounded and focused.

Visualization plays a key role too. Picture your success in Lightsaber MMA. Visualize achieving your goals. This powerful tool not only motivates you but also helps align your daily actions with your ultimate objectives. When combined with progress tracking, visualization bridges the gap between where you are and where you want to be.

Let's not forget the power of feedback in this journey. Seeking input from coaches and peers is invaluable. It provides an external perspective on your progress, offering insights that you might have missed. Constructive feedback, coupled with your tracking, fosters a holistic approach to improvement.

One effective way to track progress is by maintaining a training journal. Documenting your daily workouts, techniques practiced, and feedback received creates a tangible record of your journey. Over time, this journal becomes a testament to your dedication and growth, providing motivation and a sense of accomplishment.

In the realm of Lightsaber MMA, adaptability is key. Your progress tracking should be flexible, allowing adjustments in your training as you evolve. This flexibility ensures that your journey is not rigid but a dynamic one, adapting to your growing skills and changing goals.

Consistent progress tracking also teaches resilience. There will be days of immense progress and days when you feel stagnant. Tracking these fluctuations is crucial in developing the mental toughness required in Lightsaber MMA. It helps in understanding that progress is not always linear, and setbacks are integral to the journey.

Finally, celebrating small victories is crucial. Every milestone achieved, no matter how small, is a step towards your larger goal. Acknowledging these achievements fuels your motivation and reinforces your belief in your abilities.

In Lightsaber MMA, as in life, the path to success is a journey of continuous learning and growth. Consistent progress tracking is your ally in this journey, providing direction, motivation, and a clear perspective on your path to excellence. Keep pushing, keep tracking, and keep thriving!

Create a goal-setting plan and track your progress regularly to stay motivated and on track.

4. Engaging with the Lightsaber MMA Community

The Lightsaber MMA community is a rich source of knowledge, inspiration, and support. Engaging with this community can enhance your learning experience and provide valuable connections.

"Unlocking the Power of Community in Lightsaber MMA"

The incredible benefits of being part of the Lightsaber MMA community, both online and offline.

First and foremost, engaging in this community is about connection. Lightsaber MMA isn't just a physical activity; it's a journey that brings together people from all walks of life with a common passion. This shared interest creates a bond that goes beyond the physical aspects of the sport. Whether you're practicing in a local dojo or interacting in an online forum, the sense of belonging is profound.

Online, the community thrives through forums, social media groups, and virtual events. These platforms offer a wealth of resources - from tutorial videos to discussion threads. They are places where enthusiasts, irrespective of their geographical location, come together to share tips, experiences, and encouragement. This digital connection breaks down barriers, allowing you to be part of a global community.

Offline, the physical training sessions and events provide an unparalleled experience. Here, you engage not just with the sport but with people who share your enthusiasm. The physical presence of others creates an energetic environment that's motivating and uplifting. It's a space where you can see others in action, learn from them, and get immediate feedback on your techniques.

The community also plays a critical role in fostering personal growth. Lightsaber MMA isn't just about mastering techniques; it's about self-discovery and improvement. Being surrounded by like-minded individuals who are also on their journeys of growth and discovery can be incredibly inspiring. It creates an environment where you're encouraged to push your boundaries, experiment with new techniques, and step out of your comfort zone.

This communal setting is also a haven for developing resilience and mental toughness. Lightsaber MMA, like any martial art, comes with its challenges. There will be days when you feel like you're not making progress or when a particular move seems impossible to master. In such moments, the community becomes your support system. The encouragement and advice from fellow practitioners can turn your frustration into a learning opportunity.

Another significant benefit is the opportunity for networking and forming lasting friendships. The connections you make through Lightsaber MMA can extend beyond the sport. These can be people who support you in other areas of your life, offer professional advice, or simply become great friends.

The community also provides a platform for leadership and mentorship. As you grow in your practice, you get the opportunity to guide newcomers, share your experiences, and become a role model. This is not just rewarding but also reinforces your learning.

Lastly, let's not overlook the fun and enjoyment that comes from being part of this community. Whether it's a local meet-up or an online competition, these gatherings are filled with excitement, laughter, and shared joy. They are reminders that while the pursuit of mastery in Lightsaber MMA is serious, it is also an activity that brings joy and fulfillment.

The Lightsaber MMA community, both online and offline, is a vibrant ecosystem that offers more than just skill development. It's about connections, growth, support, and fun. It's a community that enriches your practice and, in many ways, your life.

"The Transformative Power of Community in Lightsaber MMA"

The enriching role that community engagement plays in the journey of Lightsaber MMA enthusiasts. Personal growth isn't just about the individual; it's often catalyzed by the community we immerse ourselves in.

In the world of Lightsaber MMA, community engagement is a cornerstone of training and personal development. It's not just about learning the techniques; it's about the shared experiences, the collective energy, and the support system that forms when like-minded individuals come together.

I've witnessed firsthand how joining a Lightsaber MMA community can transform an individual's training experience. One such story is of a young woman who began her Lightsaber MMA journey with hesitation and self-doubt. She struggled not just with the physical aspects of the sport but also with finding her place within it. However, once she connected with a local Lightsaber MMA group, her entire approach changed. The group's supportive environment, combined with shared experiences and encouragement, provided her with a sense of belonging and confidence. Her skills improved dramatically, but more importantly, she discovered a newfound sense of self-belief and purpose.

Another inspiring example comes from an online Lightsaber MMA forum. A man from a remote area, without access to physical training facilities, sought advice and guidance online. Through video tutorials, online workshops, and vibrant discussions on the forum, he not only honed his skills but also formed meaningful connections. The virtual community became his training ground, his source of motivation, and his gateway to diverse perspectives. His journey underscores the power of digital connections in enhancing our learning and personal growth.

Community engagement in Lightsaber MMA also fosters an environment of continuous learning and improvement. A seasoned practitioner shared how teaching beginners at his local dojo not only helped others but also refined his understanding of the sport. Through teaching, he gained new insights into Lightsaber MMA techniques and developed greater patience and empathy – skills that are invaluable both inside and outside the dojo.

The Lightsaber MMA community is also a platform for sharing triumphs and setbacks. This was evident in the story of a practitioner who faced a significant setback due to an injury. The community rallied around her, offering support, advice, and encouragement. This collective empathy and understanding played a crucial role in her recovery and return to training. Her experience highlights how community support can be a powerful force in overcoming challenges and setbacks.

The Lightsaber MMA community is much more than a group of individuals practicing the same sport. It's a dynamic, supportive, and empowering ecosystem that enriches each member's training experience. It's about shared growth, collective learning, and the bonds that form when people come together with a common passion.

"The Power of Shared Knowledge in Lightsaber MMA"

I want to talk about the incredible power of sharing knowledge, experiences, and challenges within the Lightsaber MMA community. This isn't just about martial arts; it's about the journey of growth, learning, and connection.

In the dynamic world of Lightsaber MMA, each practitioner's journey is unique, but the shared experiences bind them together. The exchange of knowledge and experiences is not just beneficial; it's crucial for personal and collective growth. Why? Because when we share, we expand our perspectives, we learn, and we grow together.

First, let's talk about the importance of sharing knowledge. Imagine a practitioner who's been training for years, mastering intricate techniques and strategies. When this individual shares their knowledge with others, it does more than just educate; it inspires and empowers. It creates a ripple effect, where one person's learning becomes a valuable resource for many. And in turn, it fosters a culture of continuous learning, where everyone, from beginners to advanced practitioners, benefits.

Then there's the aspect of sharing experiences. Lightsaber MMA isn't just a physical practice; it's a journey filled with highs and lows, triumphs and setbacks. Sharing these experiences, be it a breakthrough moment or a challenging obstacle, creates a sense of camaraderie and community. It reminds everyone that they are not alone in their journey. This connection is invaluable. It's what turns a group of individuals into a supportive community.

But it's not just about the good times; sharing challenges is equally important. When practitioners open up about the hurdles they face, it does two things: it provides an opportunity to gain insights and solutions from others, and it cultivates an environment of empathy and support. This is crucial in a discipline as challenging as Lightsaber MMA, where mental and emotional resilience are as important as physical strength.

Moreover, when practitioners share their challenges, it normalizes the struggles that come with learning something as complex as Lightsaber MMA. It breaks down the unrealistic expectation of constant perfection and progress, and it builds a more realistic, human approach to learning and growth.

The exchange of knowledge and experiences also fosters innovation and creativity. When practitioners from diverse backgrounds and skill levels come together, they bring different perspectives and ideas. This diversity is a breeding ground for new techniques, strategies, and approaches to training and combat. It's how the sport evolves and how practitioners grow not just in skill but in creativity and adaptability.

Sharing knowledge, experiences, and challenges within the Lightsaber MMA community is more than a practice; it's a powerful tool for growth, connection, and innovation. It builds a strong, supportive, and dynamic community where everyone, regardless of their level, feels valued and empowered.

Join Lightsaber MMA forums, social media groups, or local clubs to connect with other enthusiasts.

CHAPTER NINE

Fulfilling the Legacy:
The Lasting Impact of Lightsaber MMA

Leaving a Mark in the World of Martial Arts
  - Envisioning Future Landscape w/ Lightsaber MMA Integration
  - Influencing Popular Culture and Broader Societal Trends
  - Legacy and Continued Evolution of Lightsaber MMA

Subsection: Leaving a Mark in the World of Martial Arts

1. Envision the Future Landscape with Lightsaber MMA Integration

As we look ahead, the integration of Lightsaber MMA into the broader martial arts landscape is not just a possibility but a transformative reality. It represents a future where tradition meets innovation, where martial arts continue to evolve and stay relevant in a rapidly changing world.

"The Future of Martial Arts: The Impact of Lightsaber MMA"

Lightsaber MMA is not just a thrilling sport but a revolution in the world of martial arts. Imagine a future where martial arts isn't just about tradition, but also innovation, where the lines between science fiction and reality blur to create something extraordinary. That future is being shaped right now by Lightsaber MMA.

Let's talk about innovation. Lightsaber MMA is a blend of the timeless principles of martial arts with the cutting-edge excitement of science fiction. This integration is not just about the physical aspect of the sport but also about a mindset shift. Traditional martial arts focus heavily on discipline, technique, and heritage. Lightsaber MMA embraces these values while also encouraging creativity and forward-thinking. It's a symbol of how martial arts can evolve, combining respect for the past with a vision for the future.

Now, consider the impact on physical training. Lightsaber MMA requires agility, precision, and strategy – skills that are fundamental in martial arts. However, the use of a lightsaber adds a unique dimension. It demands a higher level of spatial awareness, reflexes, and hand-eye coordination. This not only enhances physical capabilities but also pushes the boundaries of what martial artists thought was possible.

Let's not forget the mental and emotional aspects. The discipline required in Lightsaber MMA is intense. It's not just about mastering the weapon but mastering the self. This form of martial arts teaches practitioners to be mindful, focused, and emotionally intelligent. These skills are invaluable, not just in the dojo but in every aspect of life.

Lightsaber MMA is paving the way for a more holistic approach to martial arts, where mental and emotional training is as crucial as physical prowess.

Furthermore, Lightsaber MMA is a symbol of inclusivity and accessibility in martial arts. It attracts a diverse group of enthusiasts, from those inspired by the sci-fi elements to traditional martial artists seeking a new challenge. This inclusivity is vital for the growth of martial arts, breaking down barriers and bringing together people from different backgrounds and skill levels.

The community aspect of Lightsaber MMA cannot be overstated. It's building a global community of practitioners who share a passion for innovation, creativity, and self-improvement. This community transcends the sport, creating networks and friendships that support and inspire its members.

Finally, let's think about the cultural impact. Lightsaber MMA is making martial arts more relevant and appealing to younger generations. It combines the excitement of a popular culture phenomenon with the deep-rooted values of martial arts. This fusion is making martial arts more accessible and interesting to a broader audience, ensuring its relevance and continuation for years to come.

Lightsaber MMA is not just a passing trend; it's a catalyst for transformation in the world of martial arts. It represents innovation, physical and mental discipline, inclusivity, community, and cultural relevance. As this sport continues to grow and evolve, it will undoubtedly shape the future of martial arts, making it more dynamic, diverse, and impactful than ever before.

"Revolutionizing Martial Arts: The Visionary Impact of Lightsaber MMA"

I want to take a moment and explore the visionary impact of Lightsaber MMA on martial arts training and philosophy. This isn't just a new sport; it's a revolution that's redefining the very essence of martial arts.

Lightsaber MMA isn't just about the physicality of martial arts; it's a fusion of technology and tradition. The use of lightsabers, inspired by science fiction, brings a new dimension to training – one that requires heightened awareness, precision, and control. This integration of technology is not just transforming how techniques are executed but also how they are learned and perfected.

Traditional martial arts are deeply rooted in ancient philosophies that emphasize discipline, respect, and self-improvement. Lightsaber MMA embraces these principles while also injecting a fresh perspective. It emphasizes adaptability, creativity, and futuristic thinking. This combination of old and new philosophies is creating a more holistic approach to martial arts, making it more relevant in the modern world.

Regarding the inclusivity and diversity that Lightsaber MMA brings to martial arts. It's a discipline that appeals to a broad audience, transcending age, gender, and cultural barriers. This inclusivity not only enriches the training experience but also ensures the longevity and relevance of martial arts in our increasingly diverse society.

Now, let's discuss the transformative impact on physical and mental training. Lightsaber MMA is not just a test of physical strength and agility but also of mental acuity and emotional intelligence. Practitioners must be strategic, intuitive, and in control of their emotions. This multidimensional training is cultivating a new breed of martial artists – ones who are as mentally and emotionally skilled as they are physically.

Lightsaber MMA is changing the face of competition in martial arts. The sport's competitive element is not just about winning but about showcasing skill, creativity, and innovation. Competitions are becoming platforms for pushing the boundaries of what's possible in martial arts, encouraging practitioners to continuously evolve and improve.

The community aspect of Lightsaber MMA cannot be overstated. It's building a global network of practitioners who share a passion for innovation and self-improvement. This community is not just about training together; it's about sharing knowledge, and experiences, and fostering a culture of continuous learning and growth.

The future impact. Lightsaber MMA is not just a trend; it's setting the stage for the future of martial arts. As technology advances, we can expect even more integration of innovative tools and techniques in training. The sport is also likely to inspire new forms of martial arts, ones that we haven't even imagined yet.

Lightsaber MMA is more than just a sport; it's a visionary movement in the world of martial arts. It's redefining training methods, philosophical approaches, and the very essence of competition. As this sport continues to evolve, it will undoubtedly leave a lasting impact on martial arts, making it more dynamic, inclusive, and relevant for future generations.

"Embracing Evolution: Transforming the Martial Arts Community and Individual Practitioners"

The martial arts community stands at the cusp of a significant transformation, thanks to innovative practices like Lightsaber MMA. This evolution is not just about adopting new techniques or tools; it's about a paradigm shift in the way martial arts are perceived, practiced, and propagated.

One of the most profound benefits of this evolution is the enhanced inclusivity and diversity it brings to the martial arts world. Traditional martial arts have sometimes been perceived as rigid, with strict adherence to age-old forms and techniques. The new wave of martial arts, however, is breaking down these barriers. It welcomes people of all ages, genders, and backgrounds, making martial arts more accessible and appealing to a broader audience. This inclusivity enriches the community, bringing in fresh perspectives and fostering a more vibrant and dynamic environment.

For individual practitioners, the benefits are equally transformative. The integration of disciplines like Lightsaber MMA into martial arts training is revolutionizing the way practitioners approach their craft. It encourages a more holistic development, focusing not just on physical prowess but also on mental agility, emotional intelligence, and spiritual growth. This comprehensive approach enhances the overall well-being of practitioners, making them not just better martial artists but more balanced individuals.

Moreover, the evolution of martial arts is fostering a culture of innovation and creativity. Practitioners are encouraged to think outside the box, to experiment, and to push the boundaries of what's possible. This culture of innovation is not just elevating the skill levels within the community but is also inspiring practitioners to apply these principles of creativity and continuous improvement in other areas of their lives.

Another key benefit is the emphasis on community and collaboration. The new wave of martial arts is not just about individual achievement; it's about building a supportive and collaborative community. Practitioners are encouraged to share their knowledge, learn from each other, and grow together. This sense of community fosters a positive environment conducive to learning and personal growth.

The technological integration in modern martial arts is also equipping practitioners with new tools and methods to enhance their training. From virtual reality simulations to advanced analytics, technology is providing practitioners with insights and experiences that were previously unimaginable. This technological advancement is not just enhancing the quality of training but is also making martial arts more engaging and enjoyable.

This evolution is redefining the very philosophy of martial arts. It's shifting the focus from martial arts being purely a means of self-defense or physical activity to a path of personal transformation and self-discovery. Practitioners are learning to apply the principles of martial arts – discipline, respect, perseverance – in their everyday lives, leading to a more fulfilling and purposeful existence.

The evolution in martial arts, exemplified by practices like Lightsaber MMA, is a boon for both the community and individual practitioners. It's making martial arts more inclusive, innovative, and holistic. As we embrace this evolution, we are not just enhancing our skills but are also embarking on a journey of personal and collective growth.

2. Influencing Popular Culture and Broader Societal Trends

Lightsaber MMA's influence extends beyond the dojo; it permeates popular culture and reflects broader societal trends. Its appeal and accessibility have the power to influence perceptions of martial arts and physical fitness in the mainstream.

Lightsaber MMA, a unique blend of martial arts and the imaginative world of science fiction is revolutionizing how society views fitness and martial arts. This innovative approach transcends traditional boundaries, offering an experience that is as mentally stimulating as it is physically invigorating.

Revolutionizing Fitness

Imagine the journey of an individual who found typical gym routines monotonous. Discovering Lightsaber MMA, they were captivated by its exhilarating blend of storytelling, physicality, and the allure of the Star Wars universe. It transformed their view of fitness from a mundane task to an adventure and a form of creative expression. This transformation highlights how fitness can be a vehicle for creativity and enjoyment, rather than just a routine task.

Empowerment and Self-Confidence

Consider the impact on someone grappling with self-esteem issues. Through Lightsaber MMA, they found not just a physical workout but a source of empowerment. The discipline built more than muscle; it nurtured confidence. This form of martial arts demonstrates how integrating cultural elements into physical training can fortify both mind and body, awakening inner strength and resilience.

Community and Shared Passion

Lightsaber MMA also fosters a strong community aspect. For many, it becomes more than just a fitness regime; it's a cultural and communal experience. Individuals from diverse backgrounds, united by their love for Star Wars and martial arts, find a sense of belonging and shared passion. The community aspect becomes a supportive network, encouraging each participant to embrace growth and celebrate their journey.

Challenging Traditional Martial Arts Stereotypes

This innovative martial art breaks stereotypes about traditional martial arts training. Its inclusive, accessible approach attracts a broad range of enthusiasts, redefining who can be a martial artist and what martial arts can entail.

Holistic Approach to Personal Development

Lightsaber MMA underscores the importance of holistic development. It combines physical training with mental focus and emotional growth, offering a way to manage stress, improve concentration, and achieve mental clarity. This holistic approach transcends the training arena, impacting various aspects of life.

Cultural Impact and Influence

The influence of Lightsaber MMA extends into popular culture, introducing a fresh narrative in fitness and martial arts. It's becoming a cultural phenomenon, inspiring various forms of media and reflecting an evolving societal perspective on fitness and martial arts.

Future Implications

Lightsaber MMA represents a future where fitness and martial arts are intertwined with storytelling and imagination. It's a comprehensive approach to personal growth and well-being, blending physical activity with the excitement of a beloved fantasy universe.

Lightsaber MMA is a movement that symbolizes empowerment, community building, and the breaking of traditional barriers. This innovative approach to martial arts and fitness is reshaping societal views, demonstrating that physical and mental discipline can be a canvas for creativity, passion, and collective growth.

In today's dynamic world, where the quest for a healthy and active lifestyle is paramount, an intriguing evolution has emerged in the realm of fitness and martial arts: Lightsaber MMA. This innovative blend of traditional martial arts and the iconic lightsaber from the Star Wars universe is not just a new form of physical exercise; it's a revolution that's captivating a wider audience, redefining fitness and wellness.

Empowering Physical Fitness

Lightsaber MMA presents a unique way to engage in physical activity. Think of it not just as a workout, but as an exhilarating adventure. This form of martial arts combines the rigorous physicality of traditional combat training with the elegance and agility of lightsaber handling, offering a full-body workout that enhances strength, flexibility, and cardiovascular health. What makes it so compelling is its ability to attract those who might have never stepped into a martial arts dojo or a gym. It breaks the monotony of traditional fitness routines, infusing energy and enthusiasm into every movement.

Mental and Emotional Well-being

Beyond the physical benefits, Lightsaber MMA plays a crucial role in mental and emotional health. It's about focus, discipline, and mindfulness. Practicing these forms, individuals find themselves immersed in a state of 'flow', where everyday stressors fade away, allowing for mental clarity and emotional balance. This aspect of Lightsaber MMA goes beyond mere physical training; it's a form of moving meditation, nurturing mental resilience and inner peace.

Community and Social Interaction

One of the most striking aspects of Lightsaber MMA is its ability to create community. Here, enthusiasts gather, not just to train, but to share a passion. This sense of belonging and shared experience fosters social connections, breaking down barriers of age, background, and fitness level. In a world where isolation is increasingly common, this communal aspect is a breath of fresh air, encouraging teamwork, camaraderie, and mutual support.

Inclusivity and Accessibility

Lightsaber MMA stands out for its inclusivity. It appeals to a broad audience – from avid Star Wars fans to those seeking an alternative fitness regime. The beauty of this martial art lies in its adaptability; it can be tailored to suit various fitness levels and abilities. This inclusivity ensures that anyone, regardless of their background in fitness or martial arts, can participate and benefit from the experience.

Cultural Impact

The cultural impact of Lightsaber MMA cannot be overstated. By bridging the gap between popular culture and physical fitness, it has introduced a novel approach to staying active. This fusion of culture and exercise has not only brought new enthusiasts into the world of martial arts but has also provided a fresh, exciting way for people to engage with a beloved franchise.

A Gateway to Lifelong Fitness

Lightsaber MMA serves as a gateway to lifelong fitness and wellness. It ignites a passion for physical activity, encouraging individuals to explore other forms of exercise and martial arts. This initial spark, kindled by the thrill of wielding a lightsaber, can lead to a sustained commitment to health and well-being.

Lightsaber MMA is a movement towards a healthier, more active lifestyle. It embodies the fusion of fun, fantasy, and fitness, resonating with a wide audience. Its impact extends beyond the physical, promoting mental well-being, community building, inclusivity, and a lasting cultural imprint. As a tool for health and happiness, Lightsaber MMA is not just transforming bodies; it's transforming lives.

3. *Legacy and Continued Evolution of Lightsaber MMA*

The legacy of Lightsaber MMA is not static; it's an ever-evolving narrative shaped by each practitioner's journey. As the discipline grows, it continues to redefine itself, embracing new challenges and opportunities for innovation.

In today's dynamic world, there's a powerful movement that's reshaping our approach to fitness and personal growth. It's called Lightsaber MMA, a fusion of the timeless discipline of martial arts with the captivating fantasy of the Star Wars universe. This isn't just a fitness trend; it's a revolution, a paradigm shift that's changing how we view exercise, mental wellness, and community.

A Bold Leap into a New Frontier of Fitness

Imagine stepping into a world where your workout is an adventure. Lightsaber MMA is that world. It's where the discipline of martial arts meets the thrill of wielding a lightsaber. This isn't just about physical fitness; it's about igniting your passion, tapping into a deeper sense of purpose, and embracing a form of exercise that speaks to your heart and soul. It's a transformative journey that goes beyond the conventional, blending excitement and discipline in a way that redefines the very essence of fitness.

Uniting People in a Shared Quest for Growth

This movement is more than a series of classes; it's the birth of a global community. It brings together people from diverse backgrounds, united by their love for a story that has touched millions and their commitment to personal growth. Here, in the heart of this community, bonds are formed, and support systems are built. It's about sharing your journey, learning from each other, and growing together. This sense of belonging, this powerful connection, is what drives the Lightsaber MMA community forward.

Transforming Lives, One Swing at a Time

Every time you pick up a lightsaber, you're not just practicing a sport; you're engaging in a full-body workout that challenges you physically and mentally. It's about agility, strength, and mental sharpness. But more than that, it's about discovering your inner strength, unlocking your potential, and stepping into a version of yourself that's brimming with confidence and vitality. This is the magic of Lightsaber MMA – it transforms lives, empowering individuals to become the best version of themselves.

An Inclusive Path to Empowerment

What makes Lightsaber MMA truly remarkable is its inclusivity. It doesn't matter who you are, where you come from, or your fitness level – there's a place for you here. It's a welcoming space where everyone is encouraged to participate, learn, and grow. This inclusivity is not just about opening doors; it's about breaking down barriers, challenging stereotypes, and creating a world where everyone can thrive.

The Cultural Phenomenon Reshaping Society

Lightsaber MMA is more than a fitness program; it's a cultural phenomenon. It's influenced movies, literature, and a wide range of products. But more importantly, it's sparked a global conversation about innovation, creativity, and the power of combining our passions with our quest for health and wellness. It's a testament to the human spirit's capacity for imagination and the desire to turn fantasy into reality.

The Future is Bright and Boundless

As we look to the future, the potential of Lightsaber MMA is limitless. It's a journey that's just beginning – a journey of continuous growth, expanding communities, and evolving experiences. This is about charting a path where fitness, fantasy, and fulfillment walk hand in hand, where every session is an opportunity to explore, learn, and transform.

Lightsaber MMA isn't just changing the way we exercise; it's revolutionizing how we connect with ourselves and each other. It's a movement that celebrates our journeys, fosters a sense of community, and inspires us to reach new heights. The legacy of Lightsaber MMA is being written every day, and it's a story of empowerment, unity, and endless possibility. Let's embrace this journey together and see where it takes us – the adventure is just beginning!

In a world that's constantly evolving, the key to not just surviving but thriving is adaptation and innovation. This principle is vividly exemplified in the realm of Lightsaber MMA, a revolutionary blend of martial arts and the captivating world of science fiction. As we delve into this dynamic field, it's crucial to understand the vital role that adaptation and innovation play in maintaining its relevance and impact.

Adaptation: The Heart of Evolution

Adaptation is about more than change; it's about evolution. In the context of Lightsaber MMA, this means continuously refining techniques, embracing new training methodologies, and being responsive to the changing needs and interests of practitioners. It's about understanding that as our society evolves, so too do our ways of learning, interacting, and staying fit. Adaptation in Lightsaber MMA isn't just about keeping pace with the times; it's about setting the pace and leading the charge into new, unexplored territories of fitness and martial arts.

Innovation: The Spark of Revolution

Innovation, on the other hand, is the spark that ignites revolution. It's what turned the ancient practice of martial arts into the thrilling spectacle of Lightsaber MMA. Innovation means looking at the lightsaber not just as a weapon in a fictional universe but as a tool for fitness, a medium for art, and a symbol of personal growth. It's about leveraging technology, such as virtual reality, to transform how we practice and experience Lightsaber MMA, making it more immersive, accessible, and engaging.

Staying Relevant in a Fast-Paced World

The world is moving faster than ever, and staying relevant is crucial. For Lightsaber MMA, this means constantly seeking new ways to connect with people's passions and interests. It's about being at the forefront of combining physical fitness with the emotional thrill of a deeply loved narrative. Staying relevant means understanding that people are looking for experiences that resonate on a deeper level, and Lightsaber MMA provides just that - a blend of physical prowess and storytelling.

Expanding Impact Through Accessibility and Inclusivity

One of the most beautiful aspects of Lightsaber MMA is its inclusivity. By continually adapting and innovating, we make this art form accessible to a wider audience. It's no longer just for those who grew up with Star Wars; it's for anyone seeking a unique way to improve their fitness, learn self-defense, or simply find a community where they belong. This expansion of impact is crucial in a world where connection and inclusivity are more important than ever.

Building a Legacy of Continuous Growth

Finally, adaptation and innovation are about building a legacy. A legacy of Lightsaber MMA that's rooted in continuous growth, pushing boundaries, and breaking new ground. It's about leaving a mark not just in the world of martial arts or fitness but in the broader narrative of how we as humans engage with our passions and pursue our health and well-being.

In conclusion, the importance of adaptation and innovation in Lightsaber MMA cannot be overstated. They are the twin engines driving this incredible journey forward, ensuring its ongoing relevance and impact. As we continue to evolve and innovate, we ensure that Lightsaber MMA remains a vibrant, dynamic, and essential part of our lives, inspiring us to reach new heights in every aspect of our being. The future is bright, and it's ours to shape.

Be an active part of the evolution by experimenting with new techniques and contributing to the Lightsaber MMA community.

ACKNOWLEDGMENTS

Writing this book has been an incredible journey, and I am deeply grateful to those who have supported and inspired me along the way.

First and foremost, I would like to thank my family for their unwavering support and understanding. To my wife, who has been my rock and my inspiration, your love and encouragement have been invaluable.

I am profoundly grateful to the dedicated students and practitioners of Light Sword Martial Arts. Your passion, commitment, and enthusiasm for lightsaber combat have been a constant source of motivation. Special thanks to those who participated in early workshops and provided invaluable feedback that shaped the techniques and principles outlined in this book.

A heartfelt thank you to my mentors and teachers in the martial arts community, who have guided me with wisdom and patience. Your teachings have laid the foundation for my growth as a martial artist and as a person.

I also want to acknowledge the creative publishing team for their hard work and dedication in bringing this book to life. Your expertise in design, editing, and publishing has been instrumental in making this project a reality.

To my friends and colleagues in the lightsaber combat community, thank you for your camaraderie and for pushing the boundaries of what is possible in martial arts. Your innovation and creativity continue to inspire me.

Finally, to all the readers and martial arts enthusiasts who embark on this journey with me, thank you for your interest and support. May this book ignite your inner warrior and inspire you to explore new horizons in the world of martial arts.

With gratitude,
Sifu Edward Armstrong

Thanks for reading! Please add a short review on Amazon or my website and let me know what you thought!

ABOUT THE AUTHOR

Sifu Armstrong is the renowned author of several books where he shares his step-by-step blueprint of how to establish a profitable career helping others understands the true power of the mind while enhancing and strengthening their own sensory perceptions and abilities.

Sifu Armstrong specializes in teaching the discoveries and tactics used to forge the unveiling of what may be considered the most innovative path towards self discovery and sensory perception enhancement.

Sifu Armstrong was awarded the Hola Awards Entrepreneur of the Year Award and the People's Choice Award. Sifu Armstrong is currently a Certified Spring Forest QiGong Specialist as well as a Board Certified Tai Chi Instructor by the Tai Chi For Health Institute.

Believing strongly in the "Henry Ford Approach" of surrounding yourself with the people who have the required skill set to get specific tasks done successfully; Sifu Armstrong purchased a European Franchise system that taught the sport of Light Saber engagements. Thus, using their Franchise systems alongside his business knowledge and experience, led to having grown this particular European Light Saber franchise organization's Largest Light Saber Dueling Academy in the United States within the first six months.

After remaining with the franchise system for two successful years and becoming a Certified Instructor for both Form 1 and Form 2 of Lightsaber Dueling.... Sifu Armstrong realized that internal changes needed to be made for light saber activities to reach their fullest potential within the United States.

With help and alliance from Friends who shared the same visions, Saberation was born.

Saberation is a National Light Saber Martial Arts, Fitness and Athletic Association that not only focuses on the disciplines of Martial Arts but the fitness and athletic aspects as well... All while using a Light Saber to both change and save lives. Saberation is also the Official Board of License and Certifications Review to all Light Sword Martial Arts Instructors and Coaches.

The City Of Virginia Beach also contracted Sifu Armstrong to provide Light Sword Martial Arts classes at various Parks & Rec Locations and has been featured on multiple media syndications and publications.

Sifu Armstrong has also been the main keynote speaker at several major conferences including the Holistic Health & Wellness Expo in Los Angeles, California where he delivered a speech on Lightsaber Movement Therapy and its physical implementations.

www.SifuArmstrong.com